Recent Advances in Dry Eye Disease

Edited by Danial Roshandel

Published in London, United Kingdom

Recent Advances in Dry Eye Disease
http://dx.doi.org/10.5772/intechopen.106300
Edited by Danial Roshandel

Contributors
Pushpa D. Rao, Hossein Aghaei, Parya Abdolalizadeh, Eduardo Rojas Alvarez, Naima Pino Urias, Rachel Dandar, John Sheppard, Danial Roshandel, Helia Ashourizadeh, Alfonso L. Sabater, Robby Mattes, Marcela Huertas-Bello

First published in London, United Kingdom, 2023 by IntechOpen
IntechOpen is the global imprint of INTECHOPEN LIMITED, registered in England and Wales, registration number: 11086078, 5 Princes Gate Court, London, SW7 2QJ, United Kingdom

British Library Cataloguing-in-Publication Data
A catalogue record for this book is available from the British Library

Additional hard and PDF copies can be obtained from orders@intechopen.com

Recent Advances in Dry Eye Disease
Edited by Danial Roshandel
p. cm.
Print ISBN 978-1-83768-807-4
Online ISBN 978-1-83768-808-1
eBook (PDF) ISBN 978-1-83768-809-8

Meet the editor

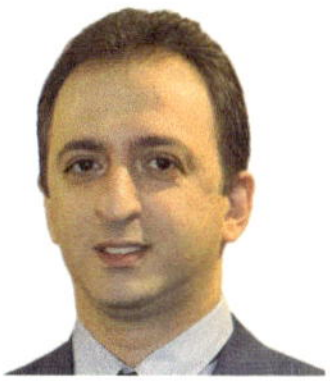

Danial Roshandel is an ophthalmologist clinician-scientist. His journey in medicine and medical research started with obtaining an MD from Golestan University of Medical Sciences, Iran, where he graduated as the top-ranked student in 2010 with experience in basic and clinical research in various fields. He completed his ophthalmology training at Shahid Beheshti University of Medical Sciences, Iran, and graduated as an eye specialist in 2014. He practiced as a general ophthalmologist specialized in ocular surface disorders for 4 years, during which he treated numerous patients with ocular surface diseases, including dry eye disease, and participated in several research projects involving patients with limbal stem cell deficiency and severe dry eye disease. In 2022, Dr. Roshandel obtained his Ph.D. in Visual Science from the University of Western Australia. He is currently a postdoctoral research fellow at the Lions Eye Institute, Perth, Australia, and an adjunct research fellow at the Centre for Ophthalmology and Visual Science, University of Western Australia. His current research projects are focused on gene therapy for inherited corneal disorders and cell-based therapies for end-stage ocular surface disorders.

Contents

Preface

Dry eye disease (DED) is one the most common ocular conditions that affects millions of individuals worldwide and poses a significant burden on patients and healthcare systems globally. Despite its prevalence, dry eye disease is often underdiagnosed and undertreated, significantly impacting the quality of life for those afflicted. Characterized by symptoms such as ocular discomfort, pain, irritation, and visual disturbances, DED results from reduced tear production, increased tear evaporation, and/or altered tear composition. In most instances, a combination of these mechanisms causes DED. The underlying causes of DED are diverse and can include age-related changes, hormonal fluctuations, environmental factors, medications, and certain systemic conditions. The growing body of research on DED has led to substantial advancements in our understanding of the pathophysiology and risk factors as well as diagnosis and management of DED. Modern lifestyle habits, such as prolonged screen time and increased exposure to air pollutants, can exacerbate DED symptoms. These discoveries have influenced patient education and led to the development of protective measures. In addition, novel diagnostic and therapeutic approaches continue to emerge and are expected to improve quality of life and result in better long-term outcomes.

Recent Advances in Dry Eye Disease is a collection of chapters authored by expert researchers and clinicians that provides an update on the mechanisms, diagnosis, and management of DED. The chapters are organized into four sections. Section 1, "Introduction", includes Chapter 1, "Introductory Chapter: Recent Advances in the Evaluation and Treatment of Dry Eye Disease ". The chapter is a summary of the risk factors that have been highlighted in recent years, especially in the era of the COVID-19 pandemic, the role of corneal imaging and tear-film parameters in the diagnosis and evaluation of DED, and clinical trials using novel treatments including artificial tear drops and topical anti-inflammatory agents. Research on the etiology of DED has continued to evolve, shedding light on new insights and potential contributing factors. In recent years, there have been advancements and emerging areas of interest. Section 2, "Updates on Etiology", provides updates on the mechanisms, risk factors, and etiology of DED in three separate chapters (Chapters 2–4). Chapter 2, "Etiology of Dry Eye ", reviews the etiologies, risk factors, and underlying mechanisms of DED. Computer vision syndrome refers to symptoms that result from prolonged use of video display terminals. It is a common condition in the modern digital age, affecting people of all ages, particularly those who spend extended periods of time in front of digital screens. In Chapter 3, "Computer Vision Syndrome", the authors review the mechanisms, manifestations, and management of computer vision syndrome. Chapter 4, "Dry Eye and Allergic Conjunctivitis", explores the mechanisms, diagnosis, and management of dry eye in patients with allergic conjunctivitis. Section 3, "Updates on Diagnosis", includes Chapter 5, "Corneal Imaging Techniques for Dry Eye Disease", which reviews the applications of conventional and modern corneal imaging techniques in the diagnosis, classification, and evaluation of DED. Novel treatments for DED aim to alleviate symptoms, improve the quality of the tear film, and promote overall ocular surface health. Intense regulated pulsed light (IRPL) therapy is a relatively new and innovative treatment option for DED. Section 4, "Updates on Management", includes Chapter 6, "Intense Regulated Pulsed Light (IRPL) for Dry Eye Treatment", in which the applications of IRPL and evidence regarding the outcomes of IRPL therapy in patients with DED have been discussed.

I would like to thank all the chapter authors for their invaluable contributions. Their expertise and dedication have enriched the content and provided readers with a comprehensive resource for staying current with the latest advancements in DED. I also express sincere appreciation to the editorial and publishing team for their support and assistance throughout the production process. Finally, I extend my gratitude to the readers of this book, including healthcare professionals, researchers, and students who seek knowledge in this field. Thank you for embarking on this journey with us, as we collectively strive to make significant advances in the understanding and management of DED.

Danial Roshandel
Centre for Ophthalmology and Visual Science,
The University of Western Australia,
Perth, Australia

Section 1

Introduction

Chapter 1

Introductory Chapter: Recent Advances in the Evaluation and Treatment of Dry Eye Disease

Danial Roshandel and Helia Ashourizadeh

1. Introduction

Dry eye disease (DED) is one of the most common ophthalmic disorders that is associated with significant vision-related, lifestyle, and economic burdens [1–3]. DED is defined as "a multifactorial disease of the ocular surface characterized by a loss of homeostasis of the tear film, and accompanied by ocular symptoms, in which tear film instability and hyperosmolarity, ocular surface inflammation and damage, and neurosensory abnormalities play etiological roles" [4]. The tear film is composed of a muco-aqueous layer protected by a lipid layer against evaporation and anchored to the corneal surface by a glycocalyx layer. Both the quantity and the quality of the tear film are important in maintaining ocular surface homeostasis [5]. Regardless of the underlying etiology, tear hyperosmolarity is the core component in the pathophysiology of the DED. It triggers a cascade of events that eventually leads to reduced expression of glycocalyx mucins, apoptotic death of surface epithelial cells, and loss of goblet cells, which in turn aggravates the hyperosmolarity state and produces a vicious circle [6]. An increase in tear osmolarity may result from decreased aqueous production, excessive evaporation, and, more commonly, a combination of both [4]. Both conditions manifest tear instability, defective tear film protection of the ocular surface, and surface damage.

The etiology, pathophysiology, diagnosis, evaluation, and treatment of DED have been studied and reviewed extensively. Due to the rapid growth of research data in this field, which has resulted in remarkable advances in understanding the risk factors, etiologies, and mechanisms of DED, along with the development of novel diagnostic and therapeutic strategies, regular updates on the recent findings and evidence are mandatory. For instance, a simple PubMed search using "dry eye disease" keyword returns more than 700 review articles (accessed on 1st May 2023), more than half of which have been published over the past 3 years.

2. Etiology and risk factors

DED is a multifactorial disorder with a complex interaction between intrinsic and extrinsic factors. Aging, hormonal changes, systemic diseases and medications, environmental conditions, contact lens wearing, eyelid abnormalities, and

IntechOpen

meibomian gland dysfunction (MGD) have been implicated in the development of DED. In recent years, factors such as lifestyle, societal, and environmental changes have been highlighted in recent studies as potential risk factors for DED that can threaten ocular surface health. In addition, the emergence of the COVID-19 pandemic and issues related to lockdowns have brought factors such as prolonged use of electronic devices and face masks and limited access to medical care during the lockdown periods to researchers' attention as important risk factors for the development and/or worsening of DED [7–10]. The impact of lifestyle changes (e.g., increased screen time and reduced outdoor activity) and environmental challenges (e.g., global warming and food insecurity) on the development, course, and management of DED requires further studies. Computer vision syndrome is another example of emerging risk factor for DED [11]. Evidence regarding the genetic predisposition to DED are limited, though further investigation can improve our understanding of the etiology and mechanisms of DED [12].

3. Diagnosis, classification, and evaluation

Diagnosis, classification, and evaluation of DED have evolved significantly over the past decade. Ancillary tests have been used extensively for diagnosing DED, determining the severity, classifying the underlying pathophysiology, and monitoring the disease course and response to therapies. Although a range of standard methods for evaluation and classification of DED has been developed and validated, newer techniques and endpoints need further investigation before they can be used in clinical trials as outcome measures. The tear film and ocular surface dry eye workshop II Diagnostic Methodology Report recommends that several factors be considered when diagnosing and evaluating DED. These factors include evaluating the symptoms and assessing the impact on vision quality. In addition, tear stability, tear volume, tear film composition, ocular surface damage, inflammation, and eyelid co-morbidities [13]. Ocular surface disease index (OSDI) and dry eye questionnaire-5 (DEQ-5) are the most common questionnaires used in clinical settings including clinical trials and are recommended by the DEWS II for the initial evaluation of dry eye symptoms. A comprehensive review of available questionnaires used in clinical studies and practice can be found in TFOS DEWS II Epidemiology Report – 2017 and a thorough review article by Okumura and colleagues [1, 14].

Numerous methods have been described to assess tear film stability. The tear film breakup time (TBUT) measures the time between a complete blink and the appearance of the first break in the tear film. TBUT is typically measured by applying fluorescein and observing the appearance of dry spots (FTBUT). An abnormal result is indicated if dry spots appear in less than 10 seconds. TBUT tests can have drawbacks such as low sensitivity and specificity, the use of fluorescein, which can affect measurements, and an invasive nature that can be uncomfortable for patients [15, 16]. Noninvasive breakup time (NIBUT) measurements have become increasingly popular in clinical practice and research due to the limitations of standard TBUT tests. Specialized equipment such as corneal topography systems, keratometers, videokeratoscopy, and interferometry-aided devices are typically used to perform these measurements [17–20].

Thermography, aberrometry, osmolarity variability, and tear evaporation rate are other methods to assess tear stability [13]. Tear evaporation is usually assessed by studies on the tear film lipid layer (TFLL) and meibomian gland structure and function. Several interferometry and thermography instruments have been introduced to measure the TFLL thickness and dynamics [21, 22]. Various methods are used to assess tear volume, including Schirmer's test without anesthesia and stimulation, which is the most popular method. Another technique to indirectly assess tear volume is strip meniscometry, which measures the lower tear meniscus volume. Tear meniscus height (TMH) can also be measured using slit-lamp bio-microscopy or digital imaging to estimate tear volume and determine aqueous deficient severity. Recently, optical coherence tomography (OCT) has emerged as a more precise method to measure tear film-related parameters. Staining of the cornea, conjunctiva, or lid margin by the fluorescein and/or Lissamine green is a reliable marker of ocular surface damage in the setting of DED. In vivo confocal microscopy [23], impression cytology [24], and ocular surface sensitivity [25] assessment are other methods to evaluate surface damage.

4. Treatment

Treatment strategies may vary depending on factors such as the type of DED (i.e., aqueous tear deficiency, evaporative tear deficiency, or combination of both), disease severity according to clinical signs (e.g., ocular surface damage) and subjective symptoms (e.g., blurred vision, pain, etc.), impact on the daily living activities and quality of life, and the underlying condition. While most mild cases can be managed by conservative measures, severe cases with a major impact on the quality of life may require a more aggressive treatment or surgical intervention.

Lubricating agents such as artificial tears are the mainstay of the treatment of DED. Numerous formulations and combinations of artificial tears are commercially available [26]. In addition, multiple new formulations and compounds are under investigation in clinical trials (e.g., NCT04701086, NCT05356728, and NCT04702776). Anti-inflammatory drops play an indispensable role in the management of moderate to severe dry eye, especially DED associated with Sjögren syndrome (SS). While corticosteroids and nonsteroidal anti-inflammatory drops such as cyclosporine and tacrolimus eye drops are being widely used for the treatment of DED in primary SS and chronic graft versus host disease [27, 28], novel agents are under investigation in various clinical trials (e.g., NCT04819269, NCT05201170 and NCT04792580).

MGD is a major cause of evaporative dry eye. Evaluation and management of MGD can be challenging. Noninvasive assessment of using in vivo confocal microscopy and anterior segment OCT can provide useful information regarding the structure and function of the meibomian glands [29]. Warm compress and lid hygiene are still the main treatments for MGD. Other methods such as intense pulsed light and vectored thermal pulsation therapy have shown promising results [30, 31].

Although conservative and medical treatments can effectively ameliorate the symptoms of DED in many patients, severe cases may require additional measures including scleral contact lenses such as prosthetic replacement of the ocular surface ecosystem [32], minimally invasive interventions such as temporary or permanent punctal occlusion [33], or more invasive surgeries such as tarsorrhaphy and salivary gland and oral mucosal grafting [34, 35]. A combination of these approaches may be used in extreme cases to prevent devastating complications such as corneal perforation.

5. Conclusion

The emergence of lifestyle, environmental, and societal risk factors and development of novel evaluation techniques and treatment strategies for DED warrants regular updates on the most recent advances and their impact on the practice pattern. The prolonged use of visual display terminals continues to be a growing concern regarding ocular surface health and can be a major risk factor for DED in the coming years. Global warming and air pollution are other potential major risk factors for DED in the future. Recent advances in the objective assessment of the tear film and meibomian glands were useful for the classification and evaluation of DED and are gaining popularity as accurate and reliable outcome measures in DED clinical trials. Similarly, artificial tear formulations have evolved notably, which may result in better ocular surface protection index and more efficient and prolonged symptom relief. In addition, novel topical anti-inflammatory drugs that selectively block immunologic responses in the ocular surface have shown promising results in clinical trials. Finally, cell and gene-based therapies may offer permanent solution for DED in certain circumstances, which requires further exploration in the future.

Author details

Danial Roshandel[1*] and Helia Ashourizadeh[2]

1 Centre for Ophthalmology and Visual Science (incorporating Lions Eye Institute), Perth, Western Australia, Australia

2 Department of Ophthalmology, Mayo Clinic, Rochester, USA

*Address all correspondence to: danial.roshandel@uwa.edu.au

References

[1] Stapleton F, Alves M, Bunya VY, Jalbert I, Lekhanont K, Malet F, et al. TFOS DEWS II epidemiology report. The Ocular Surface. 2017;**3**:334-365. DOI: 10.1016/j.jtos.2017.05.003

[2] McDonald M, Patel DA, Keith MS, Snedecor SJ. Economic and humanistic burden of dry eye disease in Europe, North America, and Asia: A systematic literature review. The Ocular Surface. 2016;**2**:144-167. DOI: 10.1016/j.jtos.2015.11.002

[3] Morthen MK, Magno MS, Utheim TP, Snieder H, Jansonius N, Hammond CJ, et al. The vision-related burden of dry eye. The Ocular Surface. 2022;**23**:207-215. DOI: 10.1016/j.jtos.2021.10.007

[4] Craig JP, Nichols KK, Akpek EK, Caffery B, Dua HS, Joo CK, et al. TFOS DEWS II definition and classification report. The Ocular Surface. 2017;**3**:276-283. DOI: 10.1016/j.jtos.2017.05.008

[5] Willcox MDP, Argueso P, Georgiev GA, Holopainen JM, Laurie GW, Millar TJ, et al. TFOS DEWS II tear film report. The Ocular Surface. 2017;**3**:366-403. DOI: 10.1016/j.jtos.2017.03.006

[6] Bron AJ, de Paiva CS, Chauhan SK, Bonini S, Gabison EE, Jain S, et al. TFOS DEWS II pathophysiology report. The Ocular Surface. 2017;**3**:438-510. DOI: 10.1016/j.jtos.2017.05.011

[7] Burgos-Blasco B, Arriola-Villalobos P, Fernandez-Vigo JI, Oribio-Quinto C, Ariño-Gutierrez M, Diaz-Valle D, et al. Face mask use and effects on the ocular surface health: A comprehensive review. The Ocular Surface. 2023;**27**:56-66. DOI: 10.1016/j.jtos.2022.12.006

[8] Galor A, Britten-Jones AC, Feng Y, Ferrari G, Goldblum D, Gupta PK, et al. TFOS lifestyle: Impact of lifestyle challenges on the ocular surface. The Ocular Surface. 2023;**28**:262-303. DOI: 10.1016/j.jtos.2023.04.008

[9] Alves M, Asbell P, Dogru M, Giannaccare G, Grau A, Gregory D, et al. TFOS lifestyle report: Impact of environmental conditions on the ocular surface. The Ocular Surface. 2023;**29**:1-52. DOI: 10.1016/j.jtos.2023.04.007

[10] Stapleton F, Abad JC, Barabino S, Burnett A, Iyer G, Lekhanont K, et al. TFOS lifestyle: Impact of societal challenges on the ocular surface. The Ocular Surface. 2023;**28**:165-199. DOI: 10.1016/j.jtos.2023.04.006

[11] Pavel IA, Bogdanici CM, Donica VC, Anton N, Savu B, Chiriac CP, et al. Computer vision syndrome: An ophthalmic pathology of the modern era. Medicina (Kaunas, Lithuania). 2023;**59**(2). DOI: 10.3390/medicina59020412

[12] Roshandel D, Semnani F, Rayati Damavandi A, Masoudi A, Baradaran-Rafii A, Watson SL, et al. Genetic predisposition to ocular surface disorders and opportunities for gene-based therapies. The Ocular Surface. 2023;**29**:150-165. DOI: 10.1016/j.jtos.2023.05.003

[13] Wolffsohn JS, Arita R, Chalmers R, Djalilian A, Dogru M, Dumbleton K, et al. TFOS DEWS II diagnostic methodology report. The Ocular Surface. 2017;**3**:539-574. DOI: 10.1016/j.jtos.2017.05.001

[14] Okumura Y, Inomata T, Iwata N, Sung J, Fujimoto K, Fujio K, et al. A review of dry eye questionnaires: Measuring patient-reported outcomes

and health-related quality of life. Diagnostics (Basel). 2020;**10**(8):559. DOI: 10.3390/diagnostics10080559

[15] Trees GR, Tomlinson A. Effect of artificial tear solutions and saline on tear film evaporation. Optometry and Vision Science. 1990;**12**:886-890. DOI: 10.1097/00006324-199012000-00002

[16] Vitali C, Moutsopoulos HM, Bombardieri S. The European Community study group on diagnostic criteria for Sjogren's syndrome. Sensitivity and specificity of tests for ocular and oral involvement in Sjogren's syndrome. Annals of the Rheumatic Diseases. 1994;**53**(10):637-647. DOI: 10.1136/ard.53.10.637

[17] Blackie CA, Solomon JD, Scaffidi RC, Greiner JV, Lemp MA, Korb DR. The relationship between dry eye symptoms and lipid layer thickness. Cornea. 2009;**7**:789-794. DOI: 10.1097/ICO.0b013e318191b870

[18] Alonso-Caneiro D, Iskander DR, Collins MJ. Tear film surface quality with soft contact lenses using dynamic-area high-speed videokeratoscopy. Eye & Contact Lens. 2009;**5**:227-231. DOI: 10.1097/ICL.0b013e3181b3350f

[19] Mengher LS, Bron AJ, Tonge SR, Gilbert DJ. A non-invasive instrument for clinical assessment of the pre-corneal tear film stability. Current Eye Research. 1985;**1**:1-7. DOI: 10.3109/02713688508999960

[20] Liu Z, Pflugfelder SC. Corneal surface regularity and the effect of artificial tears in aqueous tear deficiency. Ophthalmology. 1999;**5**:939-943. DOI: 10.1016/S0161-6420(99)00513-8

[21] Bai Y, Ngo W, Nichols JJ. Characterization of the thickness of the tear film lipid layer using high resolution microscopy. The Ocular Surface. 2019;**2**:356-359. DOI: 10.1016/j.jtos.2018.12.003

[22] Purslow C, Wolffsohn JS, Santodomingo-Rubido J. The effect of contact lens wear on dynamic ocular surface temperature. Contact Lens & Anterior Eye. 2005;**1**:29-36. DOI: 10.1016/j.clae.2004.10.001

[23] Alhatem A, Cavalcanti B, Hamrah P. In vivo confocal microscopy in dry eye disease and related conditions. Seminars in Ophthalmology. 2012;**5-6**:138-148. DOI: 10.3109/08820538.2012.711416

[24] Tole DM, McKelvie PA, Daniell M. Reliability of impression cytology for the diagnosis of ocular surface squamous neoplasia employing the biopore membrane. The British Journal of Ophthalmology. 2001;**2**:154-158. DOI: 10.1136/bjo.85.2.154

[25] Belmonte C, Nichols JJ, Cox SM, Brock JA, Begley CG, Bereiter DA, et al. TFOS DEWS II pain and sensation report. The Ocular Surface. 2017;**3**:404-437. DOI: 10.1016/j.jtos.2017.05.002

[26] Semp DA, Beeson D, Sheppard AL, Dutta D, Wolffsohn JS. Artificial tears: A systematic review. Clinical Optometry (Auckl). 2023;**15**:9-27. DOI: 10.2147/opto.S350185

[27] Shih KC, Lun CN, Jhanji V, Thong BY, Tong L. Systematic review of randomized controlled trials in the treatment of dry eye disease in Sjogren syndrome. Journal of Inflammation (London, England). 2017;**14**:26. DOI: 10.1186/s12950-017-0174-3

[28] Tappeiner C, Heiligenhaus A, Halter JP, Miserocchi E, Bandello F, Goldblum D. Challenges and concepts in the diagnosis and management of ocular

graft-versus-host disease. Frontiers in Medicine (Lausanne). 2023;**10**:1133381. DOI: 10.3389/fmed.2023.1133381

[29] Binotti WW, Bayraktutar B, Ozmen MC, Cox SM, Hamrah P. A review of imaging biomarkers of the ocular surface. Eye & Contact Lens. 2020;**46**(Suppl 2):S84-S105. DOI: 10.1097/icl.0000000000000684

[30] Jang JH, Lee K, Nam SH, Kim J, Kim JY, Tchah H, et al. Comparison of clinical outcomes between intense pulsed light therapy using two different filters in meibomian gland dysfunction: Prospective randomized study. Scientific Reports. 2023;**1**:6700. DOI: 10.1038/s41598-023-33526-z

[31] Novo-Diez A, López-Miguel A, Fernández I, Blanco-Vázquez M, Valencia-Sandonís C, Enríquez-de-Salamanca A, et al. Effect of a single vectored thermal pulsation treatment of Meibomian gland dysfunction patients under controlled environmental conditions. Scientific Reports. 2022;**1**:16761. DOI: 10.1038/s41598-022-20994-y

[32] Asghari B, Brocks D, Carrasquillo KG, Crowley E. OSDI outcomes based on patient demographic and Wear patterns in prosthetic replacement of the ocular surface ecosystem. Clinical Optometry (Auckl). 2022;**14**:1-12. DOI: 10.2147/opto.S337920

[33] Kuroda K, Toshida H, Sorita Y, Ichikawa K, Matsuzaki Y, Ohta T. Surgical punctal occlusion; combined lacrimal canaliculi cauterization and punctal suturing for severe dry eye. Journal of Ophthalmic & Vision Research. 2023;**2**:143-149. DOI: 10.18502/jovr.v18i2.13179

[34] Kate A, Deshmukh R, Donthineni PR, Sharma N, Vajpayee RB, Basu S. Management of corneal perforations in dry eye disease: Preferred practice pattern guidelines. Indian Journal of Ophthalmology. 2023;**4**:1373-1381. DOI: 10.4103/ijo.Ijo_2826_22

[35] Wakamatsu TH, Sant'Anna A, Cristovam PC, Alves VAF. Wakamatsu a and Gomes JAP: Minor salivary gland transplantation for severe dry eyes. Cornea. 2017;**36**(Suppl 1):S26-S33. DOI: 10.1097/ico.0000000000001358

Section 2

Updates on Etiology

Chapter 2

Etiology of Dry Eye

Pushpa D. Rao

Abstract

The scope of this chapter is to provide insights into the classification based on the significant factors causing dry eye. The etiological causes of dry eye have been classified broadly into two primary arms. The first arm, aqueous deficient dry eye (ADDE), illustrates malfunction of normal lacrimal secretion causing tear hyposecretion. ADDE is subdivided into Sjogren's and the non-Sjogren's syndrome. The former exclusively includes systemic autoimmune characteristics, while the latter comprises age-related disorders, genetic disorders, denervation in the lacrimal gland, and obstruction in tear secretion. The second arm, evaporative dry eye (EDE), explains the excessive loss of aqueous from the tear film despite the normal lacrimal secretion. Extrinsic EDE is with ocular surface pathology caused by vitamin A deficiency, contact lens wear, use of topical drugs with preservatives, and ocular surface diseases (allergic eye disease). The intrinsic EDE encompasses abnormalities in the meibomian lipid deficiency, low blink rate, and poor lid congruity. In brief, clinical tests to investigate the corneal epithelium integrity and the tear film have been discussed. This chapter aims to highlight the main etiologies of dry eye disease (DED) and current updates on techniques involved in diagnosing DED to help clinical practice.

Keywords: dry eye, etiology, tear film, tear hyperosmolarity, ocular surface

1. Introduction

Dry eye disease (DED) is associated with a chronic inflammatory condition of the ocular surface comprising tear hyperosmolarity and disorder of the lacrimal functional unit (LFU) [1]. LFU contains the lacrimal glands, ocular surface (cornea, conjunctiva, and meibomian glands), and the sensory and motor nerves that connect them to form an integrated system known as a "Reflex arc" [2]. LFU plays a significant role in maintaining the tear film in a regulated manner. Environmental, endocrinological, and cortical influence the functionality of LFU. Its function is to preserve the integrity of the tear film and the corneal transparency [2, 3]. There are two compartments of tears at the surface of the open eye. The first lies in the fornices and the spaces behind the lids, and the second is called the pre-ocular tears that comprise the tear menisci and the tear film. The tear film is about 3 μm thick layer [4]. The lipid layer hinders the evaporation of tear film surfaced on the top of the tear film, derived from the meibomian glands. The lacrimal gland mainly contributes to the aqueous component of the tear film lying below the surface lipid layer. The conjunctival goblet cells contribute to the mucin layer that lies over the corneal surface [5]. The mucin forms like a gel layer over the corneal surface and protects to keep up the moisture of the normal ocular surface. These three layers of the tear film help protect the exposed ocular surface from desiccation. Lacrimal secretion is at its minimum during sleep [6]. When the eyes are open in the waking state, the lacrimal secretion is determined by the sensory stimuli to increase the tear flow rate. A functional Reflex arc is the key to controlling the tear flow and maintaining the homeostasis of tear osmolarity. The Reflex arc comprises the afferent and the efferent limb, while the former is contributed from the trigeminal innervation of the ocular surface (cornea) [7]. The trigeminal neurons synapse in the superior salivatory nucleus in the brainstem. This is the nervus intermedius of the VIIth cranial nerve, carrying the region where the efferent limb of the reflex arc arises. These parasympathetic nerve fibers synapses with the other neuronal connections, help supply to the glandular tissues, and aid in their secretion function. The reflex arc functions as a "feedback loop" [2, 3] and can be influenced by humidity, airflow, temperature, and blink rate. Damage to the afferent sensory nerves or the efferent autonomic and motor nerves will lead to dysfunction in the tear-secreting glands. This causes an alteration in the function of LFU, leading to tear film instability and ocular surface disease, mainly dry eye. Inflammation in the ocular surface accompanying chronic alteration in tear secretion due to reduced corneal sensation results in tear film instability [8]. Therefore, dysfunction of LFU has been identified to be prominent in the development of various forms of dry eye. There are two major divisions of dry eye (discussed later in this chapter): 1. Aqueous-deficient dry eye and 2. Evaporative dry eye. Both lead to tear hyperosmolarity.

1.1 Ocular surface homeostasis and hyperosmolarity

Homeostasis in the ocular surface is correlated with the tear hyperosmolarity influenced by the sensory stimulation to the lacrimal gland via the LFU. In evaporative dry eye, the lacrimal gland is healthy to stimulate secretory response and compensate for the tear volume with a rise in tear osmolarity. However, this is accountable for a high-volume dry eye with increased tear secretion in patients suffering from meibomian gland dysfunction, which causes a deficiency of the tear film lipid layer [9]. On the contrary, the aqueous-deficient dry eye with dysfunction in the lacrimal gland is characterized by tear hyperosmolarity associated with low tear volume [10]. Of note, excessive reflex stimulation of the lacrimal gland may induce cytokine responses in the gland, initiating a cascade of autoantigen expression and T-cell activation with the release of inflammatory mediators into the tears [3]. "Lacrimal exhaustion" may also be induced due to intense reflex stimulation of the lacrimal gland [11].

Hyperosmolarity is regarded as the central mechanism for various forms of dry eye as a response to reduced tear flow or increased tear evaporation. Tear film instability and thinning of the tear film with excessive aqueous evaporation are the events that influence tear hyperosmolarity. Tear hyperosmolarity stimulates a sequence of inflammatory events in the ocular surface epithelium, involving NF-kB signaling and MAP kinases pathways [12] with the secretion of inflammatory cytokines (IL-1α, IL-1β, and TNF-α) and matrix metalloproteinases (e.g., MMP9) [13]. The cytokines activate inflammatory cells at the ocular surface [14], cause apoptosis of the surface epithelium, and reduced expression of glycocalyx mucins, eventually leading to the loss of goblet cells [15]. Damage to the epithelium or apoptosis is fundamental for ocular surface staining in a dry eye. Additionally, a loss of protective barrier (glycocalyx mucins) will aid in the dye (fluorescein) entry in comparison to the normal lubricated ocular surface with an intact ocular surface barrier [10]. Goblet cell loss is a phenomenon investigated in dry eye [16, 17], demonstrated by conjunctival biopsy and impression cytology that show reduced levels of the gel mucin MUC5AC [18]. Tear hyperosmolarity and inflammatory mediators in tear causes discomfort, especially during blinking, due to the loss of goblet cell mucin that helps maintain the ocular surface's lubrication. Ocular surface damage, mainly with the loss or damage to the epithelial glycocalyx, leads to insufficient lubrication, tear film instability, and progressive shortening of the tear film break-up time [19]. In the presence of a shorter break-up time, an increase in the level of hyperosmolarity is expected. Ocular surface damage, caused by osmotic stress and inflammatory events, will result in the reflex stimulation of the lacrimal gland. This is responsible for increasing the blink rate and increasing lacrimal tear secretion. Patients with meibomian gland dysfunction were diagnosed with the high-volume dry eye with increased tear secretion [9]. Experimental models suggest that intense reflex stimulation of the lacrimal gland may induce an inflammatory response in the gland. This will lead to a cascade of events, such as autoantigen expression in the gland, T-cell activation, and the release of inflammatory mediators into the tears [3, 20]. Reports have indicated to induce a state of "lacrimal exhaustion," which may need further evidence to test this hypothesis [21]. Tear Hyperosmolarity attained at the eye surface gives rise to a vicious cycle of events that results not only in symptoms and compensatory responses but also in ocular surface damage and mediating inflammatory responses. Eventually, it drives into a self-perpetuated disease.

1.2 The role of the environment in dry eye

Dry eye is susceptible to environmental conditions that can increase tear evaporation and osmolarity. These conditions may aggravate various forms of dry eye or trigger its onset in predisposed patients. The term environment can be broadly divided into (a) physiological variation between the individuals that include low natural blink rate [22], variations in the palpebral aperture [23], and sex hormones [24, 25]. (b) ambient conditions an individual encounters include environmental factors that increase tear evaporation, such as lower relative humidity, high wind velocity, air conditioning, air travel, or exposure to another artificial environment [26]. This influences tear hyperosmolarity induced by prolonged blink interval or with widened palpebral aperture, which is common during extended usage of a video display terminal, microscopy, reading, and the performance of challenging visual tasks, which reduce the blink rate or more extended periods with the eyes held up in gaze [27]. The other factors include the use of systemic drugs, which reduce lacrimal secretion, causing tear hyperosmolarity and may be listed as a risk factor for dry eye [28]. A correlation between activities of daily living the dry eye disease symptoms has been explored [29]. Awareness of such influences may allow preventative measures to be implemented.

1.3 The role of corneal sensitivity

A phenomenon of increased corneal sensory excitability was reported in dry patients [30]. This is expected to increase pain and compensatory lacrimal response in dry eye patients. Interestingly, in dry eye, morphological changes have been recorded via confocal microscopy that showed a reduction in the subbasal nerve plexus bundles in the cornea [31]. These results relate to observations made in several reports suggesting impaired corneal sensitivity in chronic dry eye disease [32]. With advancing dry eye disease, sensory loss at the ocular surface is evident, which reduces the sensory drive and stimulation to the lacrimal gland. Therefore, tear hyperosmolarity would increase with reduced lacrimal secretion, eventually leading to a fall in tear volume and tear film thickness. Furthermore, a slowing of tear film lipid layer spreading [33], with an increase in tear evaporation, is observed. Overall, ocular surface changes during dry eye are negatively affected by a reduction in corneal sensitivity and a loss of sensory drive.

2. Major etiological causes of dry eye

The leading etiological causes of dry eye have been portrayed as etiopathogenic classification developed by the subcommittee presented in the National Eye Institute (NEI) industry workshop report with a current understanding of DED (**Figure 1**).

As stated earlier in the 1995 report, the term keratoconjunctivitis sicca (KCS) is regarded as synonymous with the term dry eye. As illustrated in **Figure 1**, there are two major classes of dry eye: (1) aqueous tear-deficient dry eye (ADDE) and (2) evaporative dry eye (EDE). ADDE refers to mainly the failure of lacrimal secretion, while EDE has been subdivided to differentiate the causes that are dependent on intrinsic conditions of the eyelids and ocular surface and those that arise from extrinsic influences. It is recognized that disease initiated in one significant division may coexist with or even progress to dry eye by another considerable mechanism. This is part of a vicious cycle of interactions that can enhance the severity of dry eye. Overall, consequences of dry eye include goblet cell loss, which will contribute to loss of tear film stability, ocular surface damage and evaporative water loss, and symptoms resulting from a failure of ocular surface lubrication and inflammation.

The major groups and subgroups of dry eye are described below.

2.1 Aqueous tear-deficient dry eye (tear deficient dry eye)

Dysfunction in the lacrimal gland leads to the aqueous-deficient dry eye that reduces lacrimal tear secretion and volume [34]. Tear-deficient dry eye causes tear hyperosmolarity. Reduced lacrimal secretion may be due to 1 Sjogren syndrome, 2

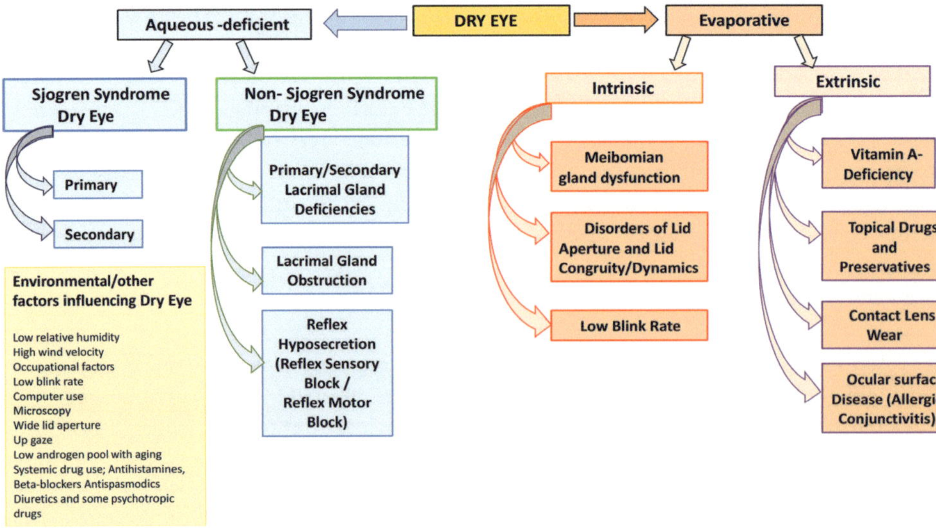

Figure 1.
Etiological classification of dry eye.

obstruction to its outflow, and 3 an intervention with the homeostatic mechanism. A reflex sensory blockade may be caused due to topical anesthesia, and efferent blockade may be due to damage in the pterygopalatine ganglion and third-order neurons [35]. Additionally, lacrimal secretion may be pharmacologically inhibited by certain systemic drugs [36]. Tear film hyperosmolarity causes an increase in osmolarity of the ocular surface epithelium and stimulates a cascade of inflammatory events involving MAP kinases and NFkB signaling pathways [12, 37] and the secretion of inflammatory cytokines (interleukin (IL)-1A; -1B; tumor necrosis factor (TNF)-A); and matrix metalloproteinases (MMP-9) [13]. During lacrimal dysfunction due to lacrimal gland infiltration and inflammation, inflammatory mediators generated in the gland may find their way into the tears and be delivered to the ocular surface. The inflammatory mediators are detected in tears and can be derived from the lacrimal gland or the ocular surface (conjunctiva and cornea). Studies have reported that the tear film lipid layer in ADDE has a delayed spreading of the lipid layer in the interblink [38, 39]. In severe ADDE, spreading may be undetectable by interferometry, suggesting significant damage to the tear film lipid layer. Delayed improper spreading of the tear film may increase an aqueous loss from the tear film. ADDE can be divided into two major subgroups, Sjogren syndrome dry eye (SSDE) and non-Sjorgen syndrome dry eye.

2.1.1 Sjogren syndrome dry eye (SSDE)

Sjogren syndrome is an exocrinopathy that involves the lacrimal and salivary glands targeted by an autoimmune process. Immune cell infiltration, mainly the activated T cells, occurs in the lacrimal and salivary glands, which causes acinar and ductular cell death. This leads to the hyposecretion of tears or saliva. The inflammatory process in the glands leads to the expression of autoantigens in the epithelium of the ocular surface [40] with the homing of tissue-specific CD4 and CD8 T-cells [41]. Th1 cells and cytokines as INF-ϒ were considered to be the main components of tissue damage, with new evidence of the major role played by Th-17 cells (T follicular (Tf), Th22, and Treg cells—the IL-17 axis) and the cytokines, especially IL-17, in the salivary and lacrimal glands [42, 43]. A neurosecretory block influences the hyposecretion of the tears due to the effects of immune cell influx and secretion of inflammatory cytokines or the presence of circulating antibodies (e.g., anti-M3 antibody) directed against muscarinic receptors within the glands [44, 45].

There are two forms of SSDE:

a. Primary SSDE consists of ADDE integrated with symptoms of dry mouth, reduced salivary secretion, and autoantibodies [46, 47].

b. Secondary SSDE consists of the features of primary SSDE along with the characteristics of an autoimmune connective disease, such as rheumatoid arthritis, systemic lupus erythematosus, Wegener's granulomatosis, primary biliary sclerosis, polyarteritis nodosa, systemic sclerosis, or mixed connective tissue disease.

It is essential to note the risk factors of SSDE, which include genetic profile [48], androgen status [49], and exposure to environmental agents. For instance, a study investigated from a mouse model of ocular HSV-1 infection showed that the lacrimal gland was affected by the immune cell influx (CD4 and CD8 T cells), causing reduced tear volume [50]. Additionally, nutritional deficiency in omega-3, Vit C, and other unsaturated fatty acids has also been reported in patients with SSDE [51]. Environmental factors causing increased evaporative water loss from the eye may trigger inflammatory events at the ocular surface via a hyperosmolar mechanism. A defective tear film lipid layer is identified to contribute to dry eye leading to evaporation [52]. This can be correlated to high rates of meibomian gland dysfunction in SSDE patients when compared to the average population [52]. Overall, the ocular dryness in SSDE is due to hyposecretion in the lacrimal glands associated with the characteristic inflammatory changes within the gland in the presence of inflammatory mediators in tears [53].

2.1.2 Non-Sjogren syndrome dry eye

Non-Sjogren syndrome dry eye is a type of ADDE caused due to lacrimal dysfunction but not with the characteristics of systemic autoimmunity; age-related dry eye is the most common. The different types of NSSDE are briefly discussed below.

2.1.2.1 Primary lacrimal gland deficiencies

i. Age-related dry eye (ARDE): A significant age-related correlation for tear evaporation, volume, flow, and osmolarity, was reported by Mathers et al. [54]. Still, no correlation was noted by Craig and Tomlinson [55] or in other reports concerning tear turnover [56] and lipid layer [57]. With increasing age in an average population, an increase in ductal pathology has been reported that may promote lacrimal gland dysfunction by its obstructive effect [58, 59]. The ductal pathology included periductal fibrosis, interacinar fibrosis, periductal blood vessel loss, and acinar cell atrophy [58, 59]. Lymphocytic immune cell infiltrates in 70% of lacrimal glands were studied and identified as the basis of fibrosis [58]. However, it appeared to be less severe when compared to Sjogren syndrome.

ii. Congenital alacrima: Congenital alacrima is reported to be a rare cause of dry eye in youth [60]. It is also part of the autosomal recessive, triple A syndrome (Allgrove syndrome), in which congenital alacrima is accompanied by achalasia of the cardia, Addison's disease, central neurodegeneration, and autonomic dysfunction [61]. It is caused by harmful mutations in the gene encoding the protein ALADIN and is involved in RNA and protein trafficking between the nucleus and cytoplasm [62, 63].

iii. Familial dysautonomia: Familial dysautonomia (Riley Day syndrome) is an autosomal recessive disorder associated with lacrimal dysfunction. Consequences include a generalized insensitivity to pain by a marked lack of emotional and reflex tearing within a multisystem condition. This is accompanied by developmental and progressive neuronal abnormality of the lacrimal gland's cervical sympathetic and parasympathetic innervations and a defective sensory innervation of the ocular surface. This affects both small myelinated (AD) and unmyelinated (C) trigeminal neurons [64, 65]. The mutation mainly affects the gene encoding an IKB kinase-associated protein.

2.1.2.2 Secondary lacrimal gland deficiencies

Inflammatory infiltration of the lacrimal gland is known to cause dysfunction in tear secretion.

i. Sarcoidosis: Lacrimal gland infiltration by sarcoid granulomata causes dry eye [66].

ii. Lymphoma: Infiltration of the lacrimal gland by lymphomatous cells causes dry eye [67].

iii. AIDS: Dry eye may be caused by T-cell infiltration in the lacrimal gland. However, in AIDS-related dry eye, unlike SSDE, CD8 suppressor cells are predominant rather than CD4 helper cells [68].

iv. Graft versus host disease (GVHD): Dry eye is a frequently observed complication of GVHD disease. It may typically occur around six months after hematopoietic stem cell transplantation. The leading cause of this is infiltration of both CD4 and CD8 T-lymphocytes, which colocalizes with antigen-presenting fibroblasts in the periductal area of the glands leading to lacrimal gland fibrosis [69, 70].

v. Lacrimal gland ablation: Dry eye may be caused by partial or complete ablation of the palpebral and/or main lacrimal gland. However, this effect can be rescued by the accessory gland and conjunctival secretion [34]. In some species (primates), it is shown that the ablation of the main lacrimal gland may reduce basal and reflex tear secretion levels but does not lead to dry eye [71].

vi. Lacrimal gland denervation: Parasympathetic denervation of the human lacrimal gland may cause dry eye [72]. As reported in some animal model experiments, it has been shown that lacrimal gland denervation causes reduced tear flow and decreased lacrimal protein secretion associated with inflammatory changes in the gland [71].

2.1.2.3 Obstruction of the lacrimal gland ducts

Obstructing the principal, palpebral, and accessory lacrimal gland ducts lead to aqueous-deficient dry eye. Additionally, deformity in the eyelid influences uneven tear film spreading. Specific conditions are discussed below.

i. Trachoma: Trachoma comprises corneal opacity leading to blindness. It is caused by tarsal and conjunctival scarring, trichiasis, and a cicatrizing meibomian gland obstruction. A dry eye may be caused resulting from lacrimal duct obstruction, lid mal-apposition, and a deficient tear film lipid layer [73].

ii. Cicatricial pemphigoid and mucous membrane pemphigoid: This is a mucocutaneous disorder characterized by skin blistering and blistering in the mucous membranes, leading to severe conjunctival scarring. Dry eye may also be caused by an obstruction in the lacrimal gland, cicatricial MGD, and/or poor lid apposition [74, 75].

iii. Erythema multiforme: This is an acute, self-limited mucocutaneous condition usually precipitated by drugs, infection, or malignancy. Dry eye may be caused due to conjunctival scarring [76].

iv. Chemical and thermal burns: Burns that are diffuse may cause much scarring to cause dry eye [46].

2.1.2.4 Reflex hyposecretion

2.1.2.4.1 Reflex sensory block

Tear secretion in the waking state is induced by trigeminal sensory input arising from the nasolacrimal passages and the eye. When the eyes are open, an increased reflex sensory drive is stimulated from the exposed ocular surface. A depletion in the sensory movement from the ocular surface may play a role in the cause of dry eye in two routes, first, by reducing reflex-induced lacrimal tear secretion and, second, by lowering the blink rate and, thereby, increasing evaporative loss [47]. It is evident from the reports that experiment conducted on the rabbit models has shown that trigeminal denervation alters the regulation of lacrimal protein secretion [77].

i. *Contact lens wear*: Extended contact lens wear has been reported to reduce sensitivity in the cornea, and this can happen in individuals who wear hard and extended-wear contact lenses. Experimental evidence from the rabbit model showed trigeminal denervation to increase tear film osmolarity and cause morphological changes in the ocular surface characteristic of dry eye [78]. When studies were conducted on patients wearing contact lenses, elevated tear osmolarity levels were recorded, leading to dry eye symptoms [79, 80]. Therefore, this has promoted to advance of LASIK surgery in patients. However, some patients' neurotrophic deficiency or neuralgic disorder was reported post-LASIK surgery [30, 81].

ii. *Diabetes:* It is evident from the research reports that diabetes mellitus has been studied as a risk factor for dry eye [82–84]. The prevalence of dry eye symptoms was evident in 18.1% of diabetics compared to 14.1% of non-diabetics in the Beaver Dam study [83, 84]. Interestingly, reports also suggested the frequency of use of ocular lubricants in people with diabetes (20.6%) when compared to non-diabetics (13.8%) [82]. This study also investigated a correlation between abnormal glycemic levels (as indicated by serum HbA1C) and frequency of ocular lubricant use. In diabetic patients, neuropathic disorders could be hypothesized to influence tear volume levels/tear secretion from the lacrimal glands. Goebbels et al. reported lower levels of reflex tears tested by the Schirmer's test in people with diabetes with no change in the basal tear flow or the tear film break-up time tested by a fluorophotometer. A study found a reduction in reflex tearing (Schirmer test) in insulin-dependent diabetics but no difference in tear film break-up time or basal tear flow by fluorophotometry [85].

iii. *Neurotrophic keratitis*: Neurotrophic keratitis is the hallmark of the herpes ocular infection, mainly involving damage to the sensory nerves in the cornea, bulbar and palpebral conjunctiva. Sensory denervation in the ocular surface will lead to characteristic features of dry eye such as tear instability, loss of mucin-secreting goblet cells, the appearance of diffuse punctate keratitis, and occurrence of ulcerative keratitis, which may lead to perforation [86, 87]. Damage to the sensory nerves results in a reduced blink rate and lacrimal secretion of tears [88]. Furthermore, it has been proposed that sensory loss in the ocular surface will lead to the loss of trophic support with the deficiency in the expression of nerve growth factor and substance P [89–92].

2.1.2.4.2 Reflex motor block

The VII cranial nerve nervus intermedius carries postganglionic, parasympathetic nerve fibers (of pterygopalatine ganglion origin) to the lacrimal gland. Significant damage to the VII cranial nerve leads to dry eye due to loss of lacrimal secretomotor function and lacrimal hyposecretion. Additionally, incomplete lid closure with multiple neuromatosis has also been reported as a characteristic of dry eye [93]. Several studies have reported a correlation between dry eye and reduced lacrimal tear secretion with systemic drug agents such as beta-blockers, antispasmodics, diuretics, and antihistamines [84]. On the contrary, no relationship was found with calcium channel blockers or cholesterol-lowering drugs [84].

2.2 Evaporative dry eye

Evaporative dry eye is caused due to increased water loss (evaporation) from the tear film in the presence of normal lacrimal secretory function. The tear film lipid layer is the main barrier to evaporation from the ocular surface. The loss of the tear film lipid layer due to meibomian gland dysfunction (MGD) is the leading cause of evaporative dry eye. Nevertheless, evaporation may also be increased by a prolonged blink interval or a widened palpebral aperture [9]. Of note, tear hyperosmolarity is also observed as an elevated characteristic feature due to evaporative water loss from the tear film. Evaporative dry eye can be distinguished further concerning the intrinsic disease affecting lid structures or dynamics or extrinsic, where the ocular surface disease occurs due to various irrelevant exposure such as topical drugs, contact lenses, and others (discussed in Section 2.2.2).

2.2.1 Intrinsic causes

2.2.1.1 Meibomian gland dysfunction (MGD)

MGD is a condition with meibomian gland dysfunction and posterior blepharitis, the leading and common cause of evaporative dry eye [94]. MGD is associated with the obstruction in the gland hindering lipid secretion. Other observations are noted in experimental models, including glandular cyst formation and meibomian duct keratinization [95, 96]. MGD can be distinguished as simple or cicatricial, primary or secondary. In simple MGD, the orifices of the gland remain located within the eyelid skin (anterior to the mucocutaneous junction). In cicatricial MGD, the orifices of the duct are drawn posteriorly onto the tarsal mucosa and the lid. This makes it incapable of delivering lipids to the tear film. Criteria for diagnosis are based on morphologic features of the gland acini and duct orifices. Methods are developed to grade the degree of MGD [97], measure the degree of gland dropout (meibography) [98, 99], and measure the levels of lipid in the lid margin reservoir (meibometry) [100]. MGD is correlated with the deficiency in the tear film lipid layer leading to an increase in tear evaporation with a higher risk of the occurrence of evaporative dry eye. An exciting finding showed the importance of meibomian lipid composition and its effect on tear film lipid layer stability. Variations in meibomian lipid composition were investigated in different individuals; for instance, one group of subjects had low levels of cholesterol esters and esters of unsaturated fatty acids, while the other group had high levels of these fractions [101]. Intriguingly, it was studied that the eyelid commensals (coagulase-negative staphylococci [CoNS], Propionibacterium acnes, and S aureus) play a role in releasing esterases, lipases fatty acids, mono- and diglycerides into the tear film [102]. The study also showed that the subjects who had a high commensal load on the eyelid margin had meibomian lipid composition rich in cholesterol when compared to the issues with low levels of cholesterol in the meibomian lipid [103]. Therefore, microbial load on the lid margin may influence the development of blepharitis.

2.2.1.2 Disorders of lid aperture and lid/globe congruity or dynamics

An increase in palpebral fissure width exposes the tear film to greater evaporation with a risk of desiccation in the ocular surface and tear hyperosmolarity [19, 104]. Desiccation of the ocular surface occurs due to poor lid apposition or lid deformity, leading to improper tear film resurfacing [19]. In Graves' disease, the effect of proptosis on exposure is compounded by lid retraction, incomplete blinking, or lid closure, by restriction of eye movements, which plays a part in tear spreading [105]. Increased ocular surface exposure and evaporation also occur in up gaze [106]. Desiccating stress in the ocular surface may also occur in the workplace through activities such as snooker, where, while aiming, the head is inclined downward, and the eyes are in the extreme up gaze [107].

2.2.1.3 Low blink rate

A complete blinking is essential to replenish the tear film by evenly distributing the aqueous tears (lacrimal glands) and lipids (from meibomian glands) over the ocular surface. Aqueous tears evaporate from the tear film during the interval between each blink. Hence, reduced or low blinking will result in dryness of the ocular surface, leading to increased evaporative loss and dry eye.

Ocular surface desiccation may be due to a reduced blink rate, which increases the blink interval time and extends the period for tear evaporation before the next blink [108, 109]. Reduced blink rate may occur during tasks involving increased concentration, especially while working at video terminals [27], with video games, at microscopes, and when the eyes are in a downgaze, as in reading. This phenomenon may also occur in the extrapyramidal disorder Parkinson's disease (PD) due to a reduction in the dopaminergic neurons of the substantia nigra [110]. Additionally, reduced reflex tearing in PD has been associated with autonomic dysfunction, considering the presence of sympathetic and peripheral parasympathetic ganglia and Lewy bodies in the substantia nigra [111]. Other contributing factors in PD include impaired meibomian oil delivery, decreased reflex tearing due to autonomic dysfunction, and the effects of androgen deficiency on the lacrimal and meibomian glands [112]. Overall, it can be summarized from these studies that there are multiple causes of dry eye in PD.

Of note, a common extrinsic risk factor for dry eye in today's world is increased digital screen time, for example, smartphone, tablet, laptop, and computer use. Studies have reported a relationship between digital screen use and dry eye, affecting the blinking dynamics and leading to ocular dryness [113]. Furthermore, a relationship between increased digital screen use and ocular surface metrics involving tear volume and tear-break-up time status has been studied, affecting the aqueous component of the tear film [114]. Blink rates during reading tasks on digital screens have been found to reduce compared to rest conditions [27, 115]. Intriguingly, reading hard-copy material also decreases the blink rate like reading on a digital screen [116, 117]. A resurgence in digital screen use during the COVID-19 pandemic led to an increased risk factor for DED in the individuals staying home with an incentive to learn, work, and socialize remotely [118].

Digital screen use is part of everyday life and is a risk factor for DED. A valid explanation to relate digital screen use and DED is the reduced blink rate and increased percentage of incomplete blinks during the digital screen. This may lead to ocular surface dryness, eventually leading to the development of DED with chronic use of the digital screen for extended periods. Hence, the prevention of DED may involve the following:

i. Deliberately blinking the eyes.

ii. Allowing natural blinking of the eyes.

iii. Incorporating environmental modifications aimed at reducing tear evaporation from the ocular surface and compensating for tear film instability.

2.2.2 Extrinsic causes

A disease of the ocular surface disorder may lead to poor surface wetting, early tear film break-up, tear hyperosmolarity, and eventually dry eye conditions. Extrinsic causes include mainly vitamin A deficiency and the effects of extensively applied topical anesthetics and preservatives. Additionally, contact lenses may be responsible for an increased risk of dry eye.

2.2.2.1 Vitamin A deficiency

Deficiency in vitamin A may cause dry eye (xerophthalmia) through a decrease in several functional conjunctival goblet cells with reduced expression of glycocalyx mucins [119]. Vitamin A is reported to be essential for both the development of goblet cells in mucous membranes and the presentation of glycocalyx mucins [119, 120]. In patients with xerophthalmia, lacrimal acinar damage is diagnosed that may have a lacrimal, aqueous tear-deficient dry eye featured with unstable tear film [121]. Vitamin A is found to be crucial for inducing mucin gene expression, mucin production, and the maintenance of mucin [122, 123]. Retinoids have been shown to play a role in regulating mucin gene expression *In-vivo*. The reports have indicated the importance of vitamin A via studies conducted in vitamin A-deficient humans and rat models. The study reported reduced conjunctival goblet cells with keratinization in the conjunctival epithelium [124]. Therefore, vitamin A deficiency is known to cause alteration in mucin production by the ocular epithelium leading to dry eye conditions.

2.2.2.2 Topical drugs and preservatives

Topical drug components can induce a toxic and inflammatory response from the ocular surface. Topical drug (eye drop) formulations with preservatives are the most common offenders, such as benzalkonium chloride (BAC). Preservative components in the eye drop cause ocular surface epithelial cell damage leading to punctate epithelial keratitis, which interferes with the tear film stability and ocular surface lubrication (surface wettability). The effects of preservative, especially BAC, in the eye drops is a significant cause of dry eye symptoms in glaucoma patients [125]. This condition was rescued by using preservative-free eye drops [125]. Using eye drops with preservatives on a long-term basis must be avoided. The use of topical anesthesia causes ocular surface drying. It reduces lacrimal secretion by lowering the sensory drive to the lacrimal gland [126] and also reduces the blink rate. Chronic use of topical anesthetics may cause neurotrophic keratitis-inducing corneal perforation [127, 128].

2.2.2.3 Contact lens wear

Contact lens wear is prominent in the developed world. There were 35 million wearers cited in the USA in the year 2000 [129]. Therefore, it is essential to study the causes of contact lens-related symptoms and intolerance experienced in the wearers. The main reason for contact lens intolerance is dryness and discomfort in the eye [130, 131]. Long-term use of contact lens wear may induce corneal epithelial changes [132] and the expression of inflammatory surface markers (HLA-DR and ICAM-1) [133]. Several studies have indicated its effect on conjunctival goblet cell density [134] and mucin expression [133, 135]. Women report dry eye symptoms more frequently than men [80]. Dry eye symptoms in contact lens wearers are associated with a higher tear osmolarity [80]. Poor lens wettability may also play a role in the increased evaporation rate.

2.2.2.4 Ocular surface disease

Reports have indicated that chronic ocular surface disease causes tear film instability with dry eye symptoms. Allergic eye disease will provide an excellent example to discuss the phenomenon of dry eye [136].

Several forms of allergic conjunctivitis can be listed as follows: (a) seasonal allergic conjunctivitis, (b) vernal keratoconjunctivitis, and (c) atopic keratoconjunctivitis. A common mechanism that occurs during allergic conjunctivitis is the exposure to antigens inducing the release of inflammatory cytokines via degranulation of IgE-primed mast cells. A Th2 response is activated first in the conjunctiva and later in the corneal epithelium. During this process, a loss of surface membrane mucins is observed with damage to the conjunctival and corneal epithelium [137]. Damage to the ocular surface with the release of inflammatory mediators will lead to allergic symptoms and reflex stimulation of the lacrimal gland. Inflammatory changes are observed in the case of vernal keratoconjunctivitis and atopic keratoconjunctivitis. Corneal surface irregularities (punctate epithelial keratitis) and conjunctival goblet cell defects can lead to tear film instability and, eventually, to dry eye symptoms in allergic eye disease. This condition may be augmented during meibomian gland dysfunction, intensifying the ocular surface drying [138]. In atopic keratoconjunctivitis, lid apposition and tear film spreading are interfered with, thus, exacerbating the dry eye.

3. Brief overview of novel diagnostic technologies for dry eye

There are several newer diagnostic techniques for dry eye. There will be a few commonly used techniques that will be highlighted in this chapter.

i. Tear osmolarity: tear hyperosmolarity is one of the major hallmarks of dry eye. A device named "Tearlab" is commercially available to measure the osmolarity of tears. A tear collection strip is designed by the Tearlab so that the capillary action can collect along the Tearlab strip. The Tearlab strip can then be inserted into the instrument to measure tear osmolarity. This test's sensitivity was better compared to traditional techniques to test dry eye, especially in mild to moderate cases. Nevertheless, it is recommended to test the tear film break-up time in severe dry eye cases.

ii. Tear film interferometry: this technique uses infrared light interference patterns to yield a tear lipid layer image. More advanced technology is available to measure the thickness of the tear lipid layer and the tear film break-up time via inbuilt software. It will benefit the patients undergoing tests using fluorescein [139, 140].

iii. Meibography: this technique is used for imaging meibomian glands via transillumination or infrared devices. However, in patients with atrophied meibomian glands, a direct clinical identification such as notching in the eyelid will be more promiscuous than using meibography [141].

4. Conclusion

This chapter has provided insights into factors associated with dry eye disease. They have been distinguished into their primary forms, aqueous deficient and evaporative dry eye. Ocular surface abnormalities and tear hyperosmolarity are both equally essential in the mechanism of dry eye. However, water loss is the common etiological factor in both forms of dry eye disease. Etiological triggers and causes outlined in this chapter form the basis for framing diagnostic and therapeutic approaches. It is essential to consider a standardized approach for diagnosing dry eye. A standard testing regimen will be good to practice that includes tests for tear film break-up time (TBUT), Schirmer test, and corneal staining status with fluorescein. More advanced testing can lead to successful treatment strategies.

Conflict of interest

The author declares no conflict of interest.

Author details

Pushpa D. Rao[1,2]

1 Department of Pharmacology and Biomarkers, PTC Therapeutics, New Jersey, USA

2 Department of Ophthalmology, Wayne State University School of Medicine, Michigan, USA

*Address all correspondence to: pdrao@med.wayne.edu; rao.pushpa@gmail.com

References

[1] Bron AJ. The Definition and Classification of Dry Eye Disease. Cham, Switzerland: Springer Nature, Springer International Publishing AG; 2015. pp. 1-19

[2] Stern ME, Beuerman RW, Fox RI, Gao J, Mircheff AK, Pflugfelder SC. The pathology of dry eye: The interaction between the ocular surface and lacrimal glands. Cornea. 1998;**17**(6):584-589. Available from: https://pubmed.ncbi.nlm.nih.gov/9820935/

[3] Stern ME, Gao J, Siemasko KF, Beuerman RW, Pflugfelder SC. The role of the lacrimal functional unit in the pathophysiology of dry eye. Experimental Eye Research. 2004;**78**(3):409-416. Available from: http://www.ncbi.nlm.nih.gov/pubmed/15106920

[4] King-Smith PE, Fink BA, Fogt N, Nichols KK, Hill RM, Wilson GS. The thickness of the human precorneal tear film: Evidence from reflection spectra | IOVS |. ARVO Journals. 2000;**41**(11):3348-3359. Available from: https://iovs.arvojournals.org/article.aspx?articleid=2123231

[5] Dartt DA. Regulation of mucin and fluid secretion by conjunctival epithelial cells. Progress in Retinal and Eye Research. 2002;**21**(6):555-576. Available from: https://pubmed.ncbi.nlm.nih.gov/12433377/

[6] Sack RA, Beaton A, Sathe S, Morris C, Willcox M, Bogart B. Towards a closed eye model of the pre-ocular tear layer. Progress in Retinal and Eye Research. 2000;**19**(6):649-668. Available from: https://pubmed.ncbi.nlm.nih.gov/11029550/

[7] Rózsa AJ, Beuerman RW. Density and organization of free nerve endings in the corneal epithelium of the rabbit. Pain. 1982;**14**(2):105-120. Available from: https://pubmed.ncbi.nlm.nih.gov/7177676/

[8] Rao P. Alterations in Ocular Surface System during the Pathogenesis of Herpes Stromal Keratitis. Wayne State University Dissertations. Detroit, Michigan: Wayne State University School of Medicine; 2019. Available from: https://digitalcommons.wayne.edu/oa_dissertations/2181

[9] Shimazaki J, Sakata M, Tsubota K. Ocular surface changes and discomfort in patients with Meibomian gland dysfunction. Archives of Ophthalmology. 1995;**113**(10):1266-1270. Available from: https://jamanetwork.com/journals/jamaophthalmology/fullarticle/641362

[10] Bron AJ, Yokoi N, Gaffney E, Tiffany JM. Predicted phenotypes of dry eye: Proposed consequences of its natural history. The Ocular Surface. 2009;**7**(2):78-92

[11] Tang NE, Zuure PL, Pardo RD, de Keizer RJ, Van Best JA. Reflex lacrimation in patients with glaucoma and healthy control subjects by Fluorophotometry | IOVS |. ARVO Journals. 2000;**41**(3):709-714. Available from: https://iovs.arvojournals.org/article.aspx?articleid=2199888

[12] Li DQ, Chen Z, Song XJ, Luo L, Pflugfelder SC. Stimulation of matrix metalloproteinases by hyperosmolarity via a JNK pathway in human corneal epithelial cells. Investigative Ophthalmology & Visual Science. 2004;**45**(12):4302-4311. Available from: https://pubmed.ncbi.nlm.nih.gov/15557436/

[13] De Paiva CS, Corrales RM, Villarreal AL, Farley WJ, Li DQ,

Stern ME, et al. Corticosteroid and doxycycline suppress MMP-9 and inflammatory cytokine expression, MAPK activation in the corneal epithelium in experimental dry eye. Experimental Eye Research. 2006;**83**(3):526-535. Available from: https://pubmed.ncbi.nlm.nih.gov/16643899/

[14] Baudouin C. The pathology of dry eye. Survey of Ophthalmology. 2001;**45**(Suppl. 2). Available from: https://pubmed.ncbi.nlm.nih.gov/11587145/

[15] Yeh S, Song XJ, Farley W, Li DQ, Stern ME, Pflugfelder SC. Apoptosis of ocular surface cells in experimentally induced dry eye. Investigative Ophthalmology & Visual Science. 2003;**44**(1):124-129. Available from: https://pubmed.ncbi.nlm.nih.gov/12506064/

[16] Kunert KS, Tisdale AS, Gipson IK. Goblet cell numbers and epithelial proliferation in the conjunctiva of patients with dry eye syndrome treated with cyclosporine. Archives of Ophthalmology (Chicago, Ill.: 1960). 2002;**120**(3):330-337. Available from: https://pubmed.ncbi.nlm.nih.gov/11879137/

[17] Brignole F, Pisella PJ, Goldschild M, De Saint JM, Goguel A, Baudouin C. Flow cytometric analysis of inflammatory markers in conjunctival epithelial cells of patients with dry eyes. Investigative Ophthalmology & Visual Science. 2000;**41**(6):1356-1363. Available from: https://pubmed.ncbi.nlm.nih.gov/10798650/

[18] Zhao H, Jumblatt JE, Wood TO, Jumblatt MM. Quantification of MUC5AC protein in human tears. Cornea. 2001;**20**(8):873-877. Available from: https://pubmed.ncbi.nlm.nih.gov/11685069/

[19] Peng CC, Cerretani C, Braun RJ, Radke CJ. Evaporation-driven instability of the precorneal tear film. Advances in Colloid and Interface Science. 2014;**206**:250-264. Available from: https://pubmed.ncbi.nlm.nih.gov/23842140/

[20] Tsubota K. Tear dynamics and dry eye. Progress in Retinal and Eye Research. 1998;**17**(4):565-596. Available from: https://pubmed.ncbi.nlm.nih.gov/9777650/

[21] Tang NEML, Zuure PL, Pardo RD, De Keizer RJW, Van Best JA. Reflex lacrimation in patients with glaucoma and healthy control subjects by fluorophotometry. Investigative Ophthalmology and Visual Science. 2000;**41**(3):709-714

[22] Doughty MJ, Naase T. Further analysis of the human spontaneous eye blink rate by a cluster analysis-based approach to categorize individuals with "normal" versus "frequent" eye blink activity. Eye & Contact Lens. 2006;**32**(6):294-299. Available from: https://pubmed.ncbi.nlm.nih.gov/17099391/

[23] Mangubat L, Luague S. Normal measurements of the palpebral fissure and the interpalpebral distance among Filipinos. Philippine Journal of Surgery and Surgical Specialties. 1966;**21**(5):304-306. Available from: https://pubmed.ncbi.nlm.nih.gov/6013482/

[24] Sullivan DA. Tearful relationships? Sex, hormones, the lacrimal gland, and aqueous-deficient dry eye. Ocular Surface. 2004;**2**(2):92-123. Available from: https://pubmed.ncbi.nlm.nih.gov/17216082/

[25] Worda C, Nepp J, Huber JC, Sator MO. Treatment of keratoconjunctivitis sicca with topical

androgen. Maturitas. 2001;**37**(3):209-212. Available from: https://pubmed.ncbi.nlm.nih.gov/11173183/

[26] Paschides CA, Stefaniotou M, Papageorgiou J, Skourtis P, Psilas K. Ocular surface and environmental changes. Acta Ophthalmologica Scandinavica. 1998;**76**(1):74-77

[27] Tsubota K, Nakamori K. Dry eyes and video display terminals. New England Journal of Medicine. 1993;**328**(8):584-584. Available from: https://pubmed.ncbi.nlm.nih.gov/8426634/

[28] Smith JA, Albenz J, Begley C, Caffery B, Nichols K, Schaumberg D, et al. The epidemiology of dry eye disease: Report of the epidemiology Subcommittee of the International dry eye WorkShop (2007). The Ocular Surface. 2007;**5**(2):93-107. Available from: https://pubmed.ncbi.nlm.nih.gov/17508117/

[29] Iyer JV, Lee SY, Tong L. The dry eye disease activity log study. Scientific World Journal. 2012;**2012**. Article ID 589875. DOI: 10.1100/2012/589875

[30] De Paiva CS, Pflugfelder SC. Corneal epitheliopathy of dry eye induces hyperesthesia to mechanical air jet stimulation. American Journal of Ophthalmology. 2004;**137**(1):109-115. Available from: https://pubmed.ncbi.nlm.nih.gov/14700652/

[31] Benítez-Del-Castillo JM, Acosta MC, Wassfi MA, Díaz-Valle D, Gegúndez JA, Fernandez C, et al. Relation between corneal innervation with confocal microscopy and corneal sensitivity with noncontact esthesiometry in patients with dry eye. Investigative Ophthalmology and Visual Science. 2007;**48**(1):173-181

[32] Xu KP, Yagi Y, Tsubota K. Decrease in corneal sensitivity and change in tear function in dry eye. Cornea. 1996;**15**(3):235-239

[33] Yokoi N, Takehisa Y, Kinoshita S. Correlation of tear lipid layer interference patterns with the diagnosis and severity of dry eye. American Journal of Ophthalmology. 1996;**122**(6):818-824

[34] Scherz W, Dohlman CH. Is the lacrimal gland dispensable? Keratoconjunctivitis sicca after lacrimal gland removal. Archives of Ophthalmology (Chicago, Ill.: 1960). 1975;**93**(4):281-283. Available from: https://pubmed.ncbi.nlm.nih.gov/1119971/

[35] Slade SG, Linberg JV, Immediata AR. Control of lacrimal secretion after sphenopalatine ganglion block. Ophthalmic Plastic and Reconstructive Surgery. 1986;**2**(2):65-70. Available from: https://pubmed.ncbi.nlm.nih.gov/3154543/

[36] Fraunfelder FT, Sciubba JJ, Mathers WD. The role of medications in causing dry eye. Journal of Ophthalmology. 2012;**2012**. Article ID 285851. DOI: 10.1155/2012/28585

[37] Luo L, Li DQ, Corrales RM, Pflugfelder SC. Hyperosmolar saline is a proinflammatory stress on the mouse ocular surface. Eye & Contact Lens. 2005;**31**(5):186-193. Available from: https://pubmed.ncbi.nlm.nih.gov/16163009/

[38] Owens H, Phillips JR. Tear spreading rates: Post-blink. Advances in Experimental Medicine and Biology. 2002;**506**(Pt B):1201-1204. Available from: https://pubmed.ncbi.nlm.nih.gov/12614052/

[39] Goto E, Tseng SCG. Differentiation of lipid tear deficiency dry eye by kinetic analysis of tear

interference images. Archives of Ophthalmology (Chicago, Ill.: 1960). 2003;**121**(2):173-180. Available from: https://pubmed.ncbi.nlm.nih.gov/12583782/

[40] Nakamura H, Kawakami A, Eguchi K. Mechanisms of autoantibody production and the relationship between autoantibodies and the clinical manifestations in Sjögren's syndrome. Translational Research. 2006;**148**(6):281-288

[41] Hayashi Y, Arakaki R, Ishimaru N. The role of caspase cascade on the development of primary Sjögren's syndrome. The Journal of Medical Investigation. 2003;**50**(1-2):32-38

[42] Alunno A, Carubbi F, Bartoloni E, Bistoni O, Caterbi S, Cipriani P, et al. Unmasking the pathogenic role of IL-17 axis in primary Sjögren's syndrome: A new era for therapeutic targeting? Autoimmunity Reviews. 2014;**13**(12):1167-1173. Available from: https://pubmed.ncbi.nlm.nih.gov/25183242/

[43] Zhang X, Volpe EA, Gandhi NB, Schaumburg CS, Siemasko KF, et al. NK Cells Promote Th-17 Mediated Corneal Barrier Disruption in Dry Eye. PLoS ONE. 2012;7(5):e36822. DOI: 10.1371/journal.pone.0036822

[44] Zoukhri D. Effect of inflammation on lacrimal gland function. Experimental Eye Research. 2006;**82**(5):885-898. Available from: https://pubmed.ncbi.nlm.nih.gov/16309672/

[45] Dawson L, Tobin A, Smith P, Gordon T. Antimuscarinic antibodies in Sjögren's syndrome: Where are we, and where are we going? Arthritis and Rheumatism. 2005;**52**(10):2984-2995. Available from: https://pubmed.ncbi.nlm.nih.gov/16200578/

[46] Lemp MA, Baudouin C, Baum J, Dogru M, Foulks GN, Kinoshita S, et al. The definition and classification of dry eye disease: Report of the definition and classification Subcommittee of the International dry eye Workshop (2007). The Ocular Surface. 2007;**5**(2):75-92

[47] Battat L, Macri A, Dursun D, Pflugfelder SC. Effects of laser in situ keratomileusis on tear production, clearance, and the ocular surface. Ophthalmology. 2001;**108**(7):1230-1235. Available from: http://www.ncbi.nlm.nih.gov/pubmed/11425680

[48] Moutsopoulos HM, Manoussakis MN. Immunopathogenesis of Sjogren's syndrome: "facts and fancy". Autoimmunity. 1989;**5**(1-2):17-24. Available from: https://pubmed.ncbi.nlm.nih.gov/2519015/

[49] Sullivan DA et al. Are women with Sjogren's syndrome androgen deficient? Journal of Rheumatology. 2003;**30**(11):2413-2419. Available from: https://pubmed.ncbi.nlm.nih.gov/?term=Are+women+with+Sjogren's++syndrome+androgen+deficient%3F

[50] Rao P, McKown RL, Laurie GW, Suvas S. Development of lacrimal gland inflammation in the mouse model of herpes stromal keratitis. Experimental Eye Research. 2019;**184**:101-106. Available from: https://pubmed.ncbi.nlm.nih.gov/31009613/

[51] Cermak JM, Papas AS, Sullivan RM, Sullivan DA. Nutrient intake in women with primary and secondary Sjögren's syndrome. European Journal of Clinical Nutrition. 2003;**57**(2):328-334

[52] Shimazaki J, Goto E, Ono M, Shimmura S, Tsubota K. Meibomian gland dysfunction in patients with Sjogren syndrome. Ophthalmology. 1998;**105**(8):1485-1488

[53] Jones DT, Monroy D, Ji Z, Atherton SS, Pflugfelder SC. Sjögren's syndrome: Cytokine and Epstein-Barr viral gene expression within the conjunctival epithelium. IOVS. 1994;**35**(9):3493-3504. Available from: https://pubmed.ncbi.nlm.nih.gov/8056525/

[54] Mathers WD, Lane JA, Bridget ZM. Tear film changes associated with normal aging. Cornea. 1996;**15**(3):229-234

[55] Craig JP, Tomlinson A. Age and gender effects on the normal tear film. Advances in Experimental Medicine and Biology. 1998;**438**:411-415. Available from: https://pubmed.ncbi.nlm.nih.gov/9634915/

[56] Sahlin S, Chen E. Evaluation of the lacrimal drainage function by the drop test. American Journal of Ophthalmology. 1996;**122**(5):701-708. Available from: https://pubmed.ncbi.nlm.nih.gov/8909211/

[57] Norn MS. Semiquantitative interference study of fatty layer of precorneal film. Acta Ophthalmologica. 1979;**57**(5):766-774

[58] Damato BE, Allan D, Murray SB, Lee WR. Senile atrophy of the human lacrimal gland: The contribution of chronic inflammatory disease. The British Journal of Ophthalmology. 1984;**68**(9):674-680. Available from: https://pubmed.ncbi.nlm.nih.gov/6331845/

[59] Obata H, Yamamoto S, Horiuchi H, Machinami R. Histopathologic study of human lacrimal gland. Statistical analysis with special reference to aging. Ophthalmology. 1995;**102**(4):678-686. Available from: https://pubmed.ncbi.nlm.nih.gov/7724184/

[60] Davidoff E, Friedman AH. Congenital alacrima. Survey of Ophthalmology. 1977;**22**(2):113-119

[61] Arya SK, Chaudhuri Z, Jain R, Nahar R, Sood S. Congenital alacrima in Pierre Robin sequence. Cornea. 2004;**23**(6):632-634. Available from: https://pubmed.ncbi.nlm.nih.gov/15257005/

[62] Brooks BP, Kleta R, Stuart C, Tuchman M, Jeong A, Stergiopoulos SG, et al. Genotypic heterogeneity and clinical phenotype in triple A syndrome: A review of the NIH experience 2000-2005. Clinical Genetics. 2005;**68**(3):215-221. Available from: https://pubmed.ncbi.nlm.nih.gov/16098009/

[63] Krumbholz M, Koehler K, Huebner A. Cellular localization of 17 natural mutant variants of ALADIN protein in triple A syndrome - shedding light on an unexpected splice mutation. Biochemistry and Cell Biology. 2006;**84**(2):243-249. Available from: https://pubmed.ncbi.nlm.nih.gov/16609705/

[64] Axelrod FB, Chelimsky GG, Weese-Mayer DE. Pediatric autonomic disorders. Pediatrics. 2006;**118**(1):309-321

[65] Gold-von Simson G, Axelrod FB. Familial dysautonomia: Update and recent advances. Current Problems in Pediatric and Adolescent Health Care. 2006;**36**(6):218-237. Available from: https://pubmed.ncbi.nlm.nih.gov/16777588/

[66] Da Silva MDSC, Campos LR. Ocular sarcoidosis. Mayo Clinic Proceedings. 2010;**85**(10):876

[67] Heath P. Ocular lymphomas. American Journal of Ophthalmology. 1949;**32**(9):1213-1223

[68] Itescu S, Brancato LJ, Buxbaum J, Gregersen PK, Rizk CC, Croxson TS, et al. A diffuse infiltrative CD8 lymphocytosis syndrome in human

immunodeficiency virus (HIV) infection: A host immune response associated with HLA-DR5. Annals of Internal Medicine. 1990;**112**(1):3-10

[69] Ogawa Y, Okamoto S, Wakui M, Watanabe R, Yamada M, Yoshino M, et al. Dry eye after haematopoietic stem cell transplantation. The British Journal of Ophthalmology. 1999;**83**(10):1125-1130

[70] Ogawa Y, Kuwana M, Yamazaki K, Mashima Y, Yamada M, Mori T, et al. Periductal area as the primary site for T-cell activation in lacrimal gland chronic graft-versus-host disease. Investigative Ophthalmology & Visual Science. 2003;**44**(5):1888-1896. Available from: https://pubmed.ncbi.nlm.nih.gov/12714620/

[71] Maitchouk DY, Beuerman RW, Ohta T, Stern M, Varnell RJ. Tear production after unilateral removal of the main lacrimal gland in squirrel monkeys. Archives of Ophthalmology (Chicago, Ill.: 1960). 2000;**118**(2):246-252. Available from: https://pubmed.ncbi.nlm.nih.gov/10676790/

[72] Whitwell J. Denervation of the lacrimal gland. The British Journal of Ophthalmology. 1958;**42**(9):518-525

[73] Guzey M, Ozardali I, Basar E, Aslan G, Satici A, Karadede S. A survey of trachoma: The histopathology and the mechanism of progressive cicatrization of eyelid tissues. Ophthalmologica. 2000;**214**(4):277-284

[74] Wang K, Seitzman G, Gonzales JA. Ocular cicatricial pemphigoid. Current Opinion in Ophthalmology. 2018;**29**(6):543-551

[75] Gipson IK, Yankauckas M, Spurr-Michaud SJ, Tisdale AS, Rinehart W. Characteristics of a glycoprotein in the ocular surface glycocalyx. Investigative Ophthalmology & Visual Science. 1992;**33**(1):218-227. Available from: http://www.ncbi.nlm.nih.gov/pubmed/1370440

[76] Power WJ, Ghoraishi M, Merayo-Lloves J, Neves RA, Foster CS. Analysis of the acute ophthalmic manifestations of the erythema multiforme/Stevens-Johnson syndrome/toxic epidermal necrolysis disease spectrum. Ophthalmology. 1995;**102**(11):1669-1676. Available from: https://pubmed.ncbi.nlm.nih.gov/9098260/

[77] Nguyen DH, Beuerman RW, Toshida H. The effects of sensory and parasympathetic denervation on the kinases and initiation factors controlling protein synthesis in the lacrimal gland. Advances in Experimental Medicine and Biology. 2002;**506**(Pt A):65-70. Available from: https://pubmed.ncbi.nlm.nih.gov/12613890/

[78] Gilbard JP, Rossi SRHK. Tear film and ocular surface changes after closure of the meibomian gland orifices in the rabbit. Ophthalmology. 1989;**96**:1180-1186

[79] Gilbard JP, Gray KL, Rossi SR. A proposed mechanism for increased tear-film osmolarity in contact lens wearers. American Journal of Ophthalmology. 1986;**102**(4):505-507. Available from: https://pubmed.ncbi.nlm.nih.gov/3766668/

[80] Nichols JJ, Sinnott LT. Tear film, contact lens, and patient-related factors associated with contact lens-related dry eye. Investigative Ophthalmology & Visual Science. 2006;**47**(4):1319-1328. Available from: https://pubmed.ncbi.nlm.nih.gov/16565363/

[81] Wilson SE. Laser in situ keratomileusis-induced (presumed)

neurotrophic epitheliopathy. Ophthalmology. 2001;**108**(6):1082-1087

[82] De Freitas GR, Ferraz GAM, Gehlen M, Skare TL. Dry eyes in patients with diabetes mellitus. Primary Care Diabetes. 2021;**15**(1):184-186

[83] Moss SE, Klein R, Klein BEK. Prevalance of and risk factors for dry eye syndrome. Archives of Ophthalmology. 2000;**118**(9):1264-1268

[84] Moss SE, Klein R, Klein BEK. Incidence of dry eye in an older population. Archives of Ophthalmology. 2004;**122**(3):369-373

[85] Dogru M, Goebbels MJ. Tear secretion and tear film function in insulin dependent diabetics (multiple letters) [10]. The British Journal of Ophthalmology. 2000;**84**(10):1210

[86] Gilbard JP, Rossi SR. Tear film and ocular surface changes in a rabbit model of neurotrophic keratitis. Ophthalmology. 1990;**97**(3):308-312. Available from: https://pubmed.ncbi.nlm.nih.gov/2336268/

[87] Cavanagh HD, Colley AM. The molecular basis of neurotrophic keratitis. Acta Ophthalmologica. 1989;**67**(192 S):115-134

[88] Heigle TJ, Pflugfelder SC. Aqueous tear production in patients with neurotrophic keratitis. Cornea. 1996;**15**(2):135-138

[89] Yamada N, Yanai R, Kawamoto K, Nagano T, Nakamura M, Inui M, et al. Promotion of corneal epithelial wound healing by a tetrapeptide (SSSR) derived from IGF-1. Investigative Ophthalmology and Visual Science. 2006;**47**(8):3286-3292

[90] Yamada N, Yanai R, Inui M, Nishida T. Sensitizing effect of substance P on corneal epithelial migration induced by IGF-1, fibronectin, or interleukin-6. Investigative Ophthalmology and Visual Science. 2005;**46**(3):833-839

[91] Lambiase A, Rama P, Bonini S, Caprioglio G, Aloe L. Topical treatment with nerve growth factor for corneal neurotrophic ulcers. The New England Journal of Medicine. 1998;**338**(17):1174-1180. Available from: http://www.ncbi.nlm.nih.gov/pubmed/9554857

[92] Nishida T, Nakamura M, Konma T, Ofuji K, Nagano K, Tanaka T, et al. Neurotrophic keratopathy—Studies on substance P and the clinical significance of corneal sensation. Nippon Ganka Gakkai Zasshi. 1997;**101**(12):948-974. Available from: https://pubmed.ncbi.nlm.nih.gov/9436358/

[93] Baum JL, Adler ME. Pheochromocytoma, medullary thyroid carcinoma, multiple mucosal neuroma: A variant of the syndrome. Archives of Ophthalmology. 1972;**87**(5):574-584

[94] Foulks GN, Bron AJ. Meibomian gland dysfunction: A clinical scheme for description, diagnosis, classification, and grading. The Ocular Surface. 2003;**1**(3):107-126

[95] Lambert R, Smith RE. Hyperkeratinization in a rabbit model of meibomian gland dysfunction. American Journal of Ophthalmology. 1988;**105**(6):703-705. Available from: https://pubmed.ncbi.nlm.nih.gov/2454028/

[96] Lambert RW, Smith RE. Effects of 13-cis-retinoic acid on the hamster meibomian gland. The Journal of Investigative Dermatology. 1989;**92**(3):321-325. Available from: https://pubmed.ncbi.nlm.nih.gov/2918239/

[97] Bron AJ, Benjamin L, Snibson GR. Meibomian gland disease. Classification

and grading of lid changes. Eye. 1991;**5**(4):395-411

[98] Mathers WD, Shields WJ, Sachdev MS, Petroll WM, Jester JV. Meibomian gland dysfunction in chronic blepharitis. Cornea. 1991;**10**(4):277-285

[99] Robin JB, Jester JV, Nobe J, Nicolaides N, Smith RE. In vivo transillumination biomicroscopy and photography of meibomian gland dysfunction. A clinical study. Ophthalmology. 1985;**92**(10):1423-1426. Available from: https://pubmed.ncbi.nlm.nih.gov/4069605/

[100] Chew CKS, Hykin PG, Jansweijer C, Dikstein S, Tiffany JM, Bron AJ. The casual level of meibomian lipids in humans. Current Eye Research. 1993;**12**(3):255-259

[101] Shine WE, McCulley JP. The role of cholesterol in chronic blepharitis. Investigative Ophthalmology and Visual Science. 1991;**32**(8):2272-2280

[102] Dougherty JM, McCulley JP. Bacterial lipases and chronic blepharitis. IOVS. 1986;**27**(4):486-491. Available from: https://pubmed.ncbi.nlm.nih.gov/3957566/

[103] Shine WE, Silvany R, McCulley JP. Relation of cholesterol-stimulated Staphylococcus aureus growth to chronic blepharitis. IOVS. 1993;**34**(7):2291-2296. Available from: https://pubmed.ncbi.nlm.nih.gov/8505210/

[104] Gilbard JP, Farris RL. Ocular surface drying and tear film osmolarity in thyroid eye disease. Acta Ophthalmologica. 1983;**61**(1):108-116. Available from: https://pubmed.ncbi.nlm.nih.gov/6687972/

[105] Yokoi N, Bron AJ, Georgiev GA. The precorneal tear film as a fluid shell: The effect of blinking and saccades on tear film distribution and dynamics. The Ocular Surface. 2014;**12**(4):252-266. Available from: https://pubmed.ncbi.nlm.nih.gov/25284771/

[106] Tsubota K, Yamada M. Tear evaporation from the ocular surface. Investigative Ophthalmology and Visual Science. 1992;**33**(10):2942-2950

[107] Tsubota K, Nakamori K. Effects of ocular surface area and blink rate on tear dynamics. Archives of Ophthalmology (Chicago, Ill.: 1960). 1995;**113**(2):155-158. Available from: https://pubmed.ncbi.nlm.nih.gov/7864746/

[108] Abelson MB, Holly FJ. A tentative mechanism for inferior punctate keratopathy. American Journal of Ophthalmology. 1977;**83**(6):866-869. Available from: https://pubmed.ncbi.nlm.nih.gov/868989/

[109] Collins MJ, Iskander DR, Saunders A, Hook S, Anthony E, Gillon R. Blinking patterns and corneal staining. Eye & Contact Lens. 2006;**32**(6):287-293

[110] Lawrence MS, Redmond DE, Elsworth JD, Taylor JR, Roth RH. The D1 receptor antagonist, SCH 23390, induces signs of parkinsonism in African green monkeys. Life Sciences. 1991;**49**(25): 229-234. Available from: https://pubmed.ncbi.nlm.nih.gov/1836030/

[111] Magalhães M, Wenning GK, Daniel SE, Quinn NP. Autonomic dysfunction in pathologically confirmed multiple system atrophy and idiopathic Parkinson's disease—A retrospective comparison. Acta Neurologica Scandinavica. 1995;**91**(2):98-102. Available from: https://pubmed.ncbi.nlm.nih.gov/7785431/

[112] Okun MS, Walter BL, McDonald WM, Tenover JL, Green J, Juncos JL, et al. Beneficial effects of testosterone replacement for the nonmotor symptoms of Parkinson disease. Archives of Neurology. 2002;**59**(11):1750-1753. Available from: https://pubmed.ncbi.nlm.nih.gov/12433262/

[113] Stapleton F, Alves M, Bunya VY, Jalbert I, Lekhanont K, Malet F, et al. TFOS DEWS II epidemiology report. The Ocular Surface. 2017;**15**(3):334-365

[114] Al-Mohtaseb Z, Schachter S, Lee BS, Garlich J, Trattler W. The relationship between dry eye disease and digital screen use. Clinical Ophthalmology. 2021;**15**:3811-3820

[115] Weygandt JJ. The influence of eye solutions on blinking and ocular comfort at rest and during work at video display terminals. Experimental Eye Research. 2007;**68**(6):663-639. Available from: https://www.sciencedirect.com/science/article/abs/pii/S001448359890656X?via%3Dihub

[116] Rodríguez MAGCEP-CM. Blink rate and incomplete blinks in six different controlled hard-copy and electronic Reading conditions. IOVS. 2015;**56**(11):6679-6685. Available from: https://iovs.arvojournals.org/article.aspx?articleid=2463760

[117] Abusharha AA. Changes in blink rate and ocular symptoms during different reading tasks. Clinical Ophthalmology. 2017;**9**:133-138. Available from: https://www.ncbi.nlm.nih.gov/pmc/articles/PMC6118863/

[118] Nagata JM, Abdel Magid HS, Gabriel KP. Screen time for children and adolescents during the coronavirus disease 2019 pandemic. Obesity (Silver Spring). 2020;**28**(9):1582-1583. Available from: https://pubmed.ncbi.nlm.nih.gov/32463530/

[119] Tei M, Spurr-Michaud SJ, Tisdale AS, Gipson IK. Vitamin A deficiency alters the expression of mucin genes by the rat ocular surface epithelium. IOVS. 2000;**41**(1):82-88. Available from: https://pubmed.ncbi.nlm.nih.gov/10634605/

[120] Hori Y, Spurr-Michaud S, Russo CL, Argüeso P, Gipson IK. Differential regulation of membrane-associated mucins in the human ocular surface epithelium. Investigative Ophthalmology & Visual Science. 2004;**45**(1):114-122. Available from: https://pubmed.ncbi.nlm.nih.gov/14691162/

[121] Sommer A, Emran N. Tear production in vitamin A-responsive xerophthalmia. American Journal of Ophthalmology. 1982;**93**(1):84-87. Available from: https://pubmed.ncbi.nlm.nih.gov/7065090/

[122] Manna B, Lund M, Ashbaugh P, Kaufman B, Bhattacharyya SN. Effect of retinoic acid on mucin gene expression in rat airways in vitro. Biochemical Journal. 1994;**297**(Pt 2):309-313. Available from: https://pubmed.ncbi.nlm.nih.gov/8297336/

[123] Jetten AM, Rearick JI, Smits HL. Regulation of differentiation of airway epithelial cells by retinoids. Biochemical Society Transactions. 1986;**14**(5):930-933. Available from: https://pubmed.ncbi.nlm.nih.gov/3781092/

[124] Tei M, Spurr-Michaud SJ, Tisdale AS, Gipson IK. Vitamin A deficiency alters the expression of mucin genes by the rat ocular surface epithelium | IOVS |. ARVO Journals. Jan 2000;**41**(1):82-88. Available from: https://iovs.arvojournals.org/article.aspx?articleid=2123077

[125] Pisella PJ, Pouliquen P, Baudouin C. Prevalence of ocular symptoms and signs with preserved and preservative free glaucoma medication. The British Journal of Ophthalmology. 2002;**86**(4):418-423

[126] Jordan A, Baum J. Basic tear flow: Does it exist? Ophthalmology. 1980;**87**(9):920-930

[127] Pharmakakis NM, Katsimpris JM, Melachrinou MP, Koliopoulos JX. Corneal complications following abuse of topical anesthetics. European Journal of Ophthalmology. 2002;**12**(5):373-378

[128] Chen HT, Chen KH, Hsu WM. Toxic keratopathy associated with abuse of low-dose anesthetic: A case report. Cornea. 2004;**23**(5):527-529. Available from: https://pubmed.ncbi.nlm.nih.gov/15220742/

[129] McMahon TT, Zadnik K. Twenty-five years of contact lenses: The impact on the cornea and ophthalmic practice. Cornea. 2000;**19**(5):730-740. Available from: https://pubmed.ncbi.nlm.nih.gov/11009325/

[130] Schlanger JL. A study of contact lens failures. Journal of the American Optometric Association. 1993;**64**(3):220-224

[131] Pritchard N, Fonn D. Dehydration, lens movement and dryness ratings of hydrogel contact lenses. Ophthalmic & Physiological Optics. 1995;**15**(4):281-286

[132] Knop E, Brewitt H. Induction of conjunctival epithelial alterations by contact lens wearing. A prospective study. German Journal of Ophthalmology. 1992;**1**(3-4):125-134 Available from: https://pubmed.ncbi.nlm.nih.gov/1483123

[133] Pisella PJ, Malet F, Lejeune S, Brignole F, Debbasch C, Bara J, et al. Ocular surface changes induced by contact lens wear. Cornea. 2001;**20**(8):820-825. Available from: https://journals.lww.com/corneajrnl/Abstract/2001/11000/Ocular_Surface_Changes_Induced_by_Contact_Lens.9.aspx

[134] Connor CG, Campbell JB, Steel SA, Burke JH. The effects of daily wear contact lenses on goblet cell density. Journal of the American Optometric Association. 1994;**65**(11):792-794

[135] Hori Y, Argüeso P, Spurr-Michaud S, Gipson IK. Mucins and contact lens wear. Cornea. 2006;**25**(2):176-181

[136] Abelson MB, Smith L, Chapin M. Ocular allergic disease: Mechanisms, disease sub-types, treatment. The Ocular Surface. 2003;**1**(3):127-149. Available from: http://www.ncbi.nlm.nih.gov/pubmed/17075644

[137] Kunert KS, Keane-Myers AM, Spurr-Michaud S, Tisdale AS. I K Gipson alteration in goblet cell numbers and mucin gene expression in a mouse model of allergic conjunctivitis. IOVS. 2001;**42**(11):2483-2489. Available from: https://pubmed.ncbi.nlm.nih.gov/11581187/

[138] Ibrahim OMA, Matsumoto Y, Dogru M, Adan ES, Wakamatsu TH, Shimazaki J, et al. In vivo confocal microscopy evaluation of meibomian gland dysfunction in atopic-keratoconjunctivitis patients. Ophthalmology. 2012;**119**(10):1961-1968. Available from: https://pubmed.ncbi.nlm.nih.gov/22717457/

[139] Eom Y, Lee JS, Kang SY, Kim HM, Song JS. Correlation between quantitative measurements of tear film lipid layer thickness and meibomian gland loss in patients with obstructive meibomian gland dysfunction and

normal controls. American Journal of Ophthalmology. 2013;**155**(6):1104-1110. Available from: https://pubmed.ncbi.nlm.nih.gov/23465270/

[140] Hosaka E, Kawamorita T, Ogasawara Y, Nakayama N, Uozato H, Shimizu K, et al. Interferometry in the evaluation of precorneal tear film thickness in dry eye. American Journal of Ophthalmology. 2011;**151**(1):18-23

[141] Pult H, Riede-Pult B. Comparison of subjective grading and objective assessment in meibography. Contact Lens Anterior Eye. 2013;**36**(1):22-27

Chapter 3

Computer Vision Syndrome

Hossein Aghaei and Parya Abdolalizadeh

Abstract

Using of computers and other video display terminals (VDTs), such as laptops, smart phones, tablets, e-readers, and even watches, are part of our everyday life and more and more users are experiencing a variety of ocular and non-ocular symptoms related to computer use. These complaints include eyestrain, tired eyes, headaches, eye irritation, eye redness, itching, blurred vision, double vision, dry eye, and neck, back, and shoulder pain as extra-ocular issues, which have been termed computer vision syndrome (CVS). Based on pieces of evidence, between 64% and 90% of computer users experience visual symptoms. Children are also affected as they spend many hours each day using digital devices with visual displays for doing schoolwork, especially after starting the COVID-19 era, playing video games, and sending and receiving text messages on cell phones. With the increased use of these electronic devices, CVS is becoming a major public health issue. Proper identification of symptoms and causative factors is necessary for the accurate diagnosis and management. There are some strategies for reducing the complaints related to prolonged use of digital screen devices.

Keywords: computer vision syndrome, video display terminal, digital eye strain, digital device, electronic device, accommodation, vergence, asthenopia, ocular surface, dry eye

1. Introduction

The use of computers and other digital electronic devices such as tablets and smartphones for both vocational and nonvocational activities including e-mail, internet search, and entertainment such as playing games is almost universal in either developed or developing societies. Computers have made life easier in terms of unlimited access to information, improved work efficiency, and ease of communication that could not have been imagined about a few decades ago.

Despite the improvement in the quality of life, more and more people have become susceptible to the worse effects of working at a computer terminal for long time.

At first, using of computer was restricted to desktop computers located in the workplace (personal computer, PC). Today's visual requirements may include viewing laptop and tablet computers, electronic book readers, smartphones, and other digital devices either in the workplace, at home, or also as a leisure activity in any location at any time. Moreover, using of digital devices is not restricted to adults. A study of over 2000 American children between 8 and 18 years of age showed that in an average day, they spend approximately 7.5 h using entertainment media, 4.5 h watching TV, 1.5 h on a computer, and over an hour playing video games [1]. Furthermore, these digital devices have now shifted into the pockets of millions of smartphone users [2]. Most smartphone owners have been reported to be adults aged from 18 to 34 years. However, next studies reported that the majority of teenagers between 14 to 18 years in the USA (87%) own smartphones [3].

The American Optometric Association defines CVS as the combination of eye and vision problems associated with the use of computers [4]. With apparently increased use of computers and its related input devices, this well-known clinical object gains significant importance. Asthenopia and symptoms related to dry eye disease are the ocular part of the syndrome. There are also musculoskeletal, dermatological, neurological, and psychological detrimental effects that are experienced in relation to the use of different types of digital devices [5].

The complaints associated with the use of computers and other electronic devices have not yet been known to cause permanent damage. However, it may result in a reduction of work accuracy and quality, which can reduce productivity. The extensive use of different types of electronic devices for various reasons desires consideration into the extent of the detrimental effect on the population.

2. Definition

The advent of computers changed human life. Today, digital display devices are required in houses, offices, and even pockets as smartphones. In 2017, about 95% of individuals aged 18–34 used handheld electronic devices such as smartphones and tablets [6]. Most of the business-related activities are also computer-based. According to the 6th European Working Conditions Survey, more than half of European workers utilize digital devices in their working [7]. The exposure to digital screen devices is not restricted to young adults, especially, after COVID-19 pandemic due to the implementation of the new public health measures such as social distancing. As the elderly people live alone in isolated circumstances during COVID-19 outbreak, these devices help them to communicate with others and stay active socially. Similarly, the children and students have used distance education or virtual leisure after COVID-19 pandemic, which led to an increase in all symptoms associated with the abuse of these devices [8].

The term computer vision syndrome (CVS), or digital eye strain, is applied collectively to a complex of visual and ocular symptoms in users of digital display devices such as computers, tablets, and smartphones. These devices have additive effects in the long term. Moreover, any activities that require extra effort for near vision in users of digital devices can enhance CVS symptoms [9]. CVS has been recognized for more than 20 years [10]. The American Optometric Association states CVS as a collection of eye and vision disorders caused by activities that strain near vision and that occur in conjunction with or during the use of computers for long hours [4]. The symptoms of CVS are classified into internal and external categories: [4, 11] Blurred vision, eye strain/fatigue, light/glare sensitivity, delay to change focal point, diplopia, and headache are internal symptoms caused by refractive, accommodative, or vergence anomalies. External symptoms include burning, itching, and tearing, which are rooted from dry eye disease. Some musculoskeletal symptoms, such as pain in the shoulders or neck, are also considered as CVS complexes [4, 12].

The CVS is usually diagnosed subjectively using self-reported questionnaires. However, subjective complaints may not be parallel with objective clinical findings, which cause over- or under-estimation of this condition [13]. Additionally, imprecise definition of CVS and considering various symptoms have led to heterogeneous results that have made it difficult to compare this health problem between populations with different characteristics. There are some validated questionnaires being developed to diagnose this syndrome, including the 17-item computer-vision symptom scale questionnaire, a six-item visual fatigue scale, and the computer vision syndrome questionnaire (CVS-Q) [14, 15].

3. Epidemiology

The CVS is the most common occupational hazard of the twenty-first century with an increasing trend [16]. It is considered a public health crisis that reduces physical and physiological well-being, employees' quality of life, occupational efficiencies, workplace productivity, and job satisfaction [4, 17, 18]. As little as 2 hours of sustained digital device usage a day is likely to develop a range of vision-related problems [9, 13, 18]. Universally, approximately 60 to 70 million individuals suffer from CVS, with 1 million new cases annually [19]. Its prevalence varies from 50% to 90% in different populations, professionals and age groups depending on demographic, environmental, and contextual factors [19–22]. The problem of CVS is extremely high in underdeveloped nations because of the inadequate accessibility and utilization of personal protective equipment, the high workload, and the restricted break time when using a computer [5, 23].

Since 2020, the COVID-19 pandemic has changed the lifestyle of the population by forcing them to follow social distancing protocols, which makes individuals more dependent on digital devices for their communication, education, daily activities, and even entertainment. Based on the strong correlation of overuse of digital devices with the prevalence and severity of CVS, it is expected that COVID-19 pandemic plays a devastative factor for this public health problem. All age groups are affected including children [21, 24], preadolescents [8], adults [25], and elderly [26]. The prevalence of CVS even rose to 80% among students due to virtual education during the lockdown period [8, 27]. Beside students, women were at higher risk for CVS during pandemic because they helped their children in virtual learning platforms [26]. Although the prevalence of CVS has shown an increasing pattern during COVID-19 pandemic, general population suffers from lack of knowledge about CVS, as well as its protective measures [28]. During pandemic, less than 10% of people are familiar with protective devices, protective guidelines for digital device use such as 20-20-20 rule, and even regular ophthalmological visits for optical correction [28]. Meanwhile, COVID-19 infection has ocular manifestations such as conjunctivitis whose additive impact on CVS remains unknown.

4. Causes and pathophysiology

Different variables have contributed to CVS. Generally, three distinct mechanisms have been identified including (1) inappropriate oculomotor responses, (2) ocular surface disease, and, (3) poor environmental conditions [29, 30]. These mechanisms can interact with each other. Moreover, there are personal factors such as age, which affect CVS through two or three mechanisms.

4.1 Inappropriate oculomotor responses

Two eyes should have efficient vergence and accommodative responses to focus on a target. If the brightness of the target is nonuniform, sustained focus needs more ocular effort. As the components of digital targets (pixels) are brighter at the center, eyes will have repeated struggles to maintain a focus on the digital screens. It makes ciliary body fatigue and the accommodative problems associated with CVS [31].

4.1.1 Vergence

Vergence is a binocular coordination to provide a single image of a visual target by merging the retinal images of two eyes. Prolonged use of digital screen devices and overexertion of the extraocular muscles can alter the ranges of vergence amplitude, horizontally, for both convergence and divergence movements [8, 32]. Therefore, the prevalence of vergence abnormalities such as convergence insufficiency increases among computer users [33]. This non-strabismic binocular dysfunction presents as an exodeviation, which causes the CVS symptoms such as asthenopia, inefficient performance of near activities, and musculoskeletal discomfort due to abnormal head posture [8, 34, 35]. On the other hand, some have proposed that exophoria at near-distance is a compensatory action for over-convergence during long-term computer use [36]. Therefore, the subjects with small amounts of exophoria may have less CVS symptoms compared to those subjects who converged accurately on the monitor for a long time.

4.1.2 Accommodation

Inappropriate accommodative responses, whether under or over-accommodation, result in eyestrain during computer using [37]. More accommodative demand leads to more accommodative fatigue. Therefore, the closer eye-screen distance in devices such as smartphones induces more accommodative fatigue and eye strain. Some subjects with symptomatic CVS also have an increased lag of accommodative response. The delay becomes more after extended viewing due to accommodative fatigue [29]. On the other hand, transient decrease in accommodative function can occur after using digital screen devices, which returns to baseline values by the end of the workday or week [33]. In other words, computer use may produce a decline in the ability to make dynamic oculomotor changes, possibly due to fatigue. Especially, patients with CVS have poor accommodative response that produces blurred vision, diplopia, myopia, and delay in the change of focus.

4.1.3 Uncorrected refractive errors

From the perspective of refractive errors, close work can induce transient myopic shifts due to accommodative effort [30, 38, 39]. This transient refractive error remains uncorrected during near-working with computer. Therefore, computer users with myopic change can complain of asthenopia [39]. Luberto et al. [39] have suggested that the temporary myopic shift can be an objective assessment parameter for evaluation of CVS fatigue. Beside transient refractive change, having baseline refractive error, particularly myopia, adds to the risk of developing CVS [24, 38, 40]. To achieve and maintain clear and single vision of targets on digital screens, the retinal image should be focused appropriately. Thus, spherical hyperopia and high myopia should be corrected [24, 29, 30]. Astigmatic errors, as low as 0.5 to 1 diopter, are also important to increase symptoms of CVS [29]. In presbyopia, an insufficient addition in near correction makes the patient to tilt the neck backward (extension) to see the screen clearly [41]. This inappropriate posture can increase CVS symptoms. Progressive additive lenses, especially occupational types, provide good vision at near and intermediate distances for computer workers with presbyopia, which can influence both ocular symptomatology and the neck posture [42, 43].

4.1.4 Eyeglasses

Those who wear eyeglasses have a higher prevalence of CVS [9, 27, 44]. Incorrect prescriptions may cause under-correction of refractive errors, especially in individuals with presbyopia who require close proximity to the device to keep the images in focus. Indeed, computer screens are formed by pixels instead of solid images, which make focusing harder [44].

4.1.5 Contact lens

Wearing contact lenses increases the severity of ocular discomfort in patients with CVS [45, 46]. Contact lenses irritate the ocular surface, make unstable tear film, and alter the blink rate. Therefore, contact lens comfort of computer users is highly dependent on lubrication of the eye. Moreover, lens type is a key factor in the development of these symptoms. Silicone hydrogel lenses are more preferred than conventional hydrogel lenses by computer users [47]. Residual refractive errors, especially astigmatism, may also contribute to CVS among contact lens users. It is a routine practice pattern that spherical contact lenses are prescribed for subjects with astigmatism <1.0 D. Therefore, increased CVS symptoms occur, not as a result of the contact lens inducing dry eye, but rather as a result of the uncorrected refractive error.

4.2 Ocular surface disease

Decompensation and desiccation of ocular surfaces are common in computer users, which are related to corneal dryness, reduced blink rate, and increased corneal exposure.

4.2.1 Ocular and systemic disease

The likelihood of CVS is higher among computer users with a previous ocular disease either chronic or acute with long-term side effects [5, 9]. Underlying dry eye is the most important ocular disease in developing CVS among computer users. Any several systemic disease or medications contributing to ocular drying can also enhance CVS.

4.2.2 Blink rate and pattern

Normal blinking rate is 22 blinks per minute while relaxed. Using a computer over a long period alters the pattern and rate of blinking [48]. The blink rate is significantly decreased during using digital screen devices. It decreased to 10 and 7 blinks per minute during reading a book and computer texts, respectively [48]. This reduction is more as font size and contrast decrease or the cognitive demand of the task increases [49]. Additionally, the downward movement of upper eyelid is not complete during computer use. Therefore, the upper eyelid does not touch lower eyelid and does not cover exposed cornea, which causes an incomplete blinking pattern. Infrequent and incomplete blinking contributes to a poor tear film quality, insufficient wetting of the ocular surface, and temporary stresses the cornea, resulting in symptoms of dry eye.

4.2.3 Line of sight (angle of gaze)

People usually have small angle of gaze and look downwards when they read texts on the paper. In small angle of gaze, the upper eyelid covers a substantial portion of the cornea, thus preventing tear evaporation and ocular discomfort symptoms [48, 50]. On the contrary, computer users usually view the digital screens in a horizontal gaze with a wider palpebral fissure. More corneal exposure accelerates tear film instability and CVS. Angle of gaze can also alter the accommodative and vergence response, and therefore the level of CVS symptoms [51].

4.3 Poor environmental conditions

Poor ergonomic conditions and worse posture in front of digital screen devices can cause musculoskeletal symptoms. Poor lighting, imbalance of light between the computer screen and working room, and poor contrast can exacerbate CVS severity [52, 53].

4.3.1 Lighting condition

The appropriate lighting levels vary according to the tasks. Writing and reading need higher lightening levels because they are tasks with greater visual demands [54, 55]. Improper environmental lighting levels, whether low or high intensities, adversely affect ocular comfort during using computers [29, 30, 41, 56]. The weak lighting condition can cause the eyes to tire gradually [29, 41, 56]. In dark environment, blink rate is decreased that accelerates desiccation of cornea. On the other hand, bright light sources (overhead fluorescent, large windows, and desk lamps) appear to significantly reduce the accommodation amplitude, wash out screen character images, and create reflection and glare [29, 56, 57]. Nowadays, the brightness of digital screens can be adjusted according to environmental lightning levels, which provides better performance for users.

4.3.2 Workplace air conditions

The office air conditioning can influence ocular surface of computer users. A low ambient humidity, a high temperature, and ventilation fans increase the evaporation of tear film, which accelerates ocular dryness [58]. The humidity of 45% has been recommended as a lower limit for workplaces [59]. Air pollution, such as airborne paper dust, laser and photocopy toner, and building contaminants, can also affect the comfort of computer users in office, negatively [58, 60].

4.3.3 Seating position

The inappropriate seating position of computer users is associated with CVS [9, 41]. Unfortunately, the ergonomic practices are not usually applied by most of the computer users [40]. The incorrect posture causes ocular discomfort, glare, and muscular spasm. Moreover, short eye-digital screen distance exposes users to more electromagnetic radiation emitting from the computer. On the other hand, the visual demands due to poor ocular accommodation and/or under-corrected refractive errors can also result in inappropriate posture leading to musculoskeletal difficulties. Oculomotor fatigue may change the innervation to the postural muscles in the neck, shoulder, and upper back, resulting in discomfort in these areas.

4.3.4 Distance

Each type of digital screen device has its own recommended viewing distance. Eye-screen distance is 50–70 cm for computers and 20–30 cm for mobile phones and tablets with smaller screens [48, 61]. Maintaining a proper viewing distance from digital screens decreases the symptoms of CVS [20, 40]. Closer eyes to digital screens require more accommodative effort and ocular muscle stress [5, 20]. In addition, more ocular surface decompensation and exacerbation of dry eye occur in proximity of eyes to digital screens [62].

4.3.5 Time

The symptoms of CVS appear to increase as the duration of exposure increases [5, 8, 9, 20, 21, 24, 44]. This may be because a computer generates electromagnetic radiation or high-energy blue light, which stresses the ciliary muscle in the eye, resulting in eye strain after continued exposure to the computer screen. Beside the amount of daily hours, the years of computer use also affect CVS development [5]. The CVS appears to have a cumulative nature rather than to be an acute condition. Therefore, long years of using a device equal more accumulated stress on the eyes, which might intensify the risk of developing CVS.

4.3.6 Rest break

Taking rest break is a protective factor for CVS [44, 63]. Dividing the work hours by short rest times during continuous computer work results in relaxing intraocular muscles, which can then decrease eye strain and headache [18]. Additionally, tear film is refreshed during rest break.

4.3.7 Personal factors

4.3.7.1 Sex

Females display a significantly greater number of CVS symptoms [5, 11, 40–42]. This association with sex could be related to dry eye [64]. Nevertheless, some symptoms may be more frequent in males such as burning sensation, dry eyes, red eyes, and blurred vision [44].

4.3.7.2 Aging

By aging, the quality of retinal image has been decreasing due to the decrease of lens transparency, which increases the ocular aberrations and light scattering. Additionally, presbyopia is an important factor associated with asthenopia. Presbyopic digital device users experience more accommodative stress during focusing at near distance [10]. The prevalence of dry eye and ocular surface disease, as contributor factors of dry eye, are also higher among older people. However, some protective mechanisms, such as senile miosis counteract with this process, improve the depth of focus and reduce accommodative strain in elderly.

4.3.7.3 Socioeconomic level

Occupational factors such as monthly income, employment status, and job stress or exhaustion affect the prevalence of CVS [65, 66]. High-paid workers are able to afford the protective facilities such as antiglare devices, eyeglasses as well as ocular medications and lubricants. These subjects may also have better workplace conditions and good awareness on computer ergonomics [65]. In general, there is a reverse relationship between knowledge on safety measures of computer use and the severity of CVS among computer workers [65].

4.3.7.4 Multiple digital device usage

The use of digital screen devices outside work is an important factor of CVS [20, 24]. Some possible reasons may be smaller screens of smartphones and tablets, closer eye-screen distance, and longer exposure times, which aggravate the risk of experiencing CVS.

5. Ocular signs and symptoms of CVS

The most common ocular and non-ocular complaints associated with CVS or digital eyestrain are:

- Eyestrain
- Eye fatigue
- Ocular pain
- Blurred vision
- Double vision
- Dry eyes
- Stinging
- Itching
- Red eyes

Symptom category	Symptoms	Possible causes
Asthenopic	Eye strain Tired eyes Sore eyes	Binocular vision Accommodation
Ocular surface related	Dry eyes Watery eyes Irritated eyes Contact lens problems	Infrequent blinking
Visual	Blurred vision Slowness of focus change Double vision Presbyopia Transient blindness	Refractive error Accommodation Binocular vision Presbyopic correction Bleaching of photopigment, with the viewing eye becoming light-adapted
Extraocular	Neck pain Back pain Shoulder pain	Computer screen location

Table 1.
Major categories of symptoms in computer vision syndrome.

- Headache
- Neck and shoulder pain

We can put these complaints in four categories (**Table 1**).

In most occasions, symptoms of CVS occur because the visual demands of the task are more than the visual abilities of the individual to comfortably perform them. In a review of asthenopia, Sheedy et al. detected that symptoms commonly associated with this syndrome incorporated eyestrain, eye fatigue, discomfort, burning, irritation, pain, ache, sore eyes, diplopia, photophobia, blur, itching, tearing, dryness, and foreign body sensation. While investigating the effect of several symptom-inducing conditions on asthenopia, the authors determined that two vast categories of symptoms existed. The first group, termed external symptoms, included burning, irritation, ocular dryness, and tearing and was related to dry eye. The second group, termed internal symptoms, included eyestrain, headache, eye ache, diplopia, and blur and is generally caused by refractive, accommodative, or vergence anomalies. Consequently, the authors proposed that the underlying problem could be detected by the location and/or description of symptoms [67].

There are some investigations that compared visual problems in using digital devices and hard copy, and it is very interesting that even when using a modern flat panel monitor; subjects reported significantly greater blur during the computer task (increasing the demands placed upon ocular accommodation and vergence), when compared with a hard-copy printout of the same material and environmental conditions [68, 69]. Many of the visual symptoms experienced by users are only transient and will decline after stopping computer work or use of the digital device and in rare occasions it persists.

CVS, or digital eyestrain, can be diagnosed through a comprehensive eye examination. We should pay attention to patient history, visual acuity measurements, refraction, accommodation, and binocular vision status. Prolonged VDTs usage has been shown to cause reduced power of accommodation, removal of the near point of convergence, and deviation of phoria for near vision [70].

6. Treatment

Certainly, the management of CVS requires a multidirectional approach because of the variety of complaints between users. When treating a patient, it is essential to consider both ocular therapies, as well as adjustment of the user's workstation, environment, and habits in an ergo-ophthalmologic approach.

Potential therapeutic interventions for patients with symptoms of CVS can be divided into three main parts namely:

1. Refractive and accommodative disorders.

2. Vergence anomalies.

3. Ocular surface problems.

In examining patients with CVS, the following clinical parameters should be evaluated [with all near testing being performed at the distance(s) at which the electronic screen(s) are positioned]:

1. Best corrected visual acuity.

2. Refractive error (including binocular balancing)

3. Accommodative error (lag) at the appropriate working distance.

4. Monocular and binocular amplitude of accommodation.

5. Monocular and binocular accommodative facility.

6. Negative and positive relative accommodation.

When examining patients with CVS, the following clinical vergence parameters should be measured [with all near testing being performed at the distance(s) at which the electronic screen(s) are positioned]:

1. Near point of convergence.

2. Near heterophoria.

3. Horizontal and vertical fixation disparity and/or associated phoria.

4. Vergence facility.

5. Vergence ranges (negative and positive relative vergence)

6. Stereopsis.

7. AC/A and CA/C ratios.

Computer use has been associated with both a reduced rate of blinking and a high number of incomplete blinks when compared with viewing hard-copy materials. Dry eye therapies, which have been proposed to minimize symptoms of CVS, include the use of lubricating drops, ointments, and topical medications for blepharitis or allergic conditions. Additionally, blink training to increase the blink rate during computer use [71], as well as changes in ambient humidity (around 45%), hydration (drinking more water) and redirection of heating and air conditioning vents have all been proposed.

Some important points in preventing or reducing the complaints of CVS have to do with the computer and how it is used. This includes lighting conditions, chair comfort, location of reference materials, the position of the monitor, and the use of rest breaks. American optometric association has given some recommendations for proper body position during using computer, which emphasize on proper height of the chair, table, and monitor for straight position of the neck and back, as well as 90-degree angle of elbow. Moreover, a support for the feet can prevent hanging of the legs (**Figure 1**) [72].

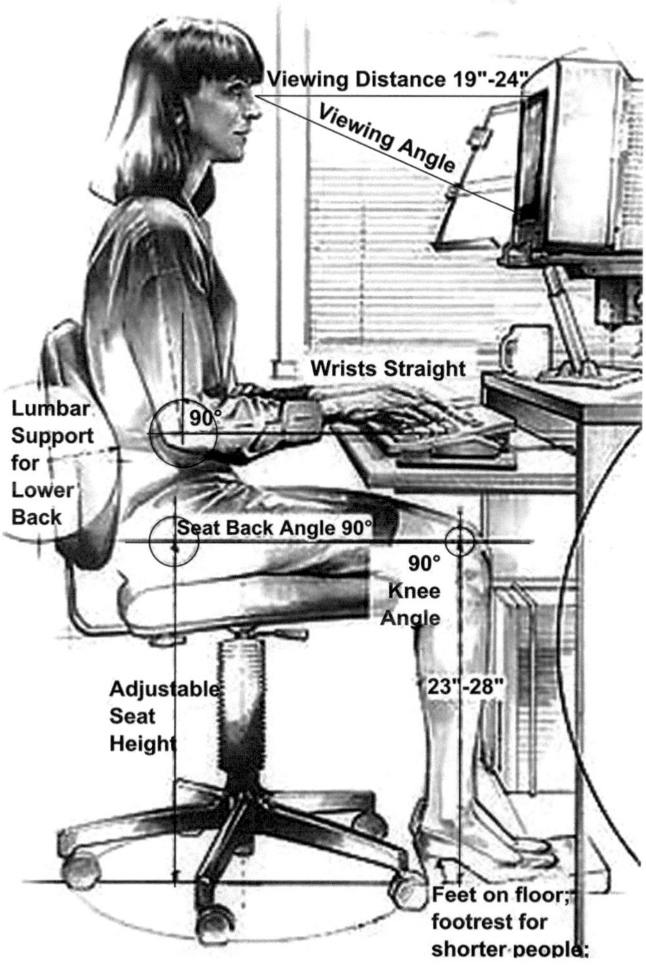

Figure 1.
Proper body positioning for computer use. Yamavu, CC0, via Wikimedia commons.

6.1 Location of the computer screen

Most people find it more comfortable to view a computer when their eyes are looking downward. Ideally, the computer screen should be 15 to 20 degrees below eye level (about 4 or 5 inches) as measured from the center of the screen and 20 to 28 inches from the eyes. This position reduces the width of palpebral fissure and consequently decreases the evaporation of tear.

6.2 Reference materials

These materials should be located above the keyboard and below the monitor. If this is not possible, a document holder can be used beside the monitor. The aim is to position the documents, so the head does not need to be repositioned from the document to the screen.

6.3 Lighting

Position the computer screen to avoid glare, particularly from overhead lighting or windows. Use blinds or drapes on windows and replace the light bulbs in desk lamps with bulbs of lower wattage.

6.4 Anti-glare screens

If there is no way to minimize glare from light sources, consider using a screen glare filter. These filters lessened the amount of light reflected from the screen.

6.5 Seating position

Chairs should be comfortably padded and conform to the body. Chair height should be adjusted so the feet rest flat on the floor. Arms should be adjusted to provide support, while typing and wrists should not rest on the keyboard when typing.

6.6 Rest breaks

To prevent eyestrain, try to rest eyes when using the computer for extended period of time. Resting the eyes for 15 minutes after 2 hours of continuous computer use. Also, for every 20 minutes of computer viewing, look into the distance 20 feet away for 20 seconds to allow the eyes a chance to refocus (20:20:20 rule).

6.7 Blinking

To minimize the chances of developing dry eye when using a computer, try to blink frequently and completely. Surface of the eye is moistened by regular and effective blinking.

7. Prevention

In providing an appropriate form of spectacle correction, practitioners must consider both the viewing distance and gaze angle (both horizontal and vertical). A mild glasses prescription may be needed to reduce vision stress on the job. It has a good idea for computer users to get a complete eye exam every year. If glasses are worn for distant vision, reading or both, they may not provide the most efficient vision for viewing a computer screen, which is about 20 to 30 inches from the eyes. Tell the doctor about job tasks and measure on-the-job sight distances. Accurate information will help get the best vision improvement. Patients may benefit from one of the new lens designs made, specifically for computer work.

Blue light from LED and fluorescent lighting, as well as monitors, tablets, and mobile devices, can negatively affect vision over the long term. Special lens tints and coatings can diminish the harmful effect of blue light. Minimize glare on the computer screen by using a glare reduction filter, repositioning the screen, or using drapes, shades, or blinds. Also, keeping screens clean, dirt-free and removing fingerprints can decrease glare and improve clarity.

7.1 Adjust work area and computer for comfort

In terms of viewing distance, the United States Occupational Safety and Health Administration state that the preferred viewing distance for a desktop monitor is between 50 and 100 cm (representing an accommodative stimulus in a corrected individual of between 1 and 2D). Additionally, they recommend that the center of the computer monitor should normally be located 15–20° below the horizontal eye level, and the entire visual area of the display screen should be located so the downward viewing angle is never >60° [73]. When using computers, most people prefer a work surface height of about 26 inches. Desks and tables are usually 29 inches high.

7.2 Use an adjustable copyholder

Place reference material at the same distance from eyes as the computer screen and as near to the screen as possible. That way the eyes will not have to change focus when looking from one to the other.

7.3 Take alternative task breaks throughout the day

Make phone calls or photocopies. Consult with coworkers. After working on the computer for an extended period, do anything in which the eyes do not have to focus on something up close.

7.4 Limit screen time for using electronic devices in children

Recommended amount of screen time for children (the Canadian Pediatric Society and the American Academy of Pediatrics):

- Infants and Toddlers (0–2 years): **None**, with the possible exception of live chatting, for example,. with grandparents.

- Preschool children (2–5 years): No more than 1 hour per day of age-appropriate.

- School-age children (5–18 years): Ideally, no more than 2 hours per day of recreational screen.

Using of special apps. Such as Microsoft's "Night light," Apple's "Night shift," and Samsung-blue Light Filter.

Adequate work environments. Appropriate room temperature (20–22°C), ambient humidity (around 45%), and no direct horizontal or upper air from ventilation fans.

Regular breaks during digital display. Take a break from the screen every 30–60 minutes is mandatory. The use of screens should be avoided 1 hour before bedtime.

Encourage outdoor activity over screen time.

8. Conclusion

Although the use of computer and other electronic devices are an inevitable part of modern life, every user should have sufficient knowledge about causes, prevention, and treatment of the visual and nonvisual side effects of long-term use of these devices. Otherwise, we have to wait for a big epidemic of visual problems, especially in children and young people, in the not-so-distant future.

Conflict of interest

The authors declare no conflict of interest.

Acronyms and Abbreviations

CVS Computer vision syndrome
VDT video display terminals

Author details

Hossein Aghaei* and Parya Abdolalizadeh
Eye Research Center, The Five Senses Institute, Rassoul Akram Hospital, Iran University of Medical Sciences, Tehran, Iran

*Address all correspondence to: draghaei.h@gmail.com

References

[1] Rideout VJ, Foehr UG, Roberts DF. Generation M2. Media in the Lives of 8- to 18-Year Olds. A Kaiser Family Foundation Study. The Henry J. Menlo Park: Kaiser Family Foundation; 2010

[2] Parihar JK, Jain VK, Chaturvedi P, Kaushik J, Jain G, Parihar AK. Computer and visual display terminals (VDT) vision syndrome (CVDTS). Medical Journal, Armed Forces India. 2016;**72**(3):270-276. DOI: 10.1016/j.mjafi.2016.03.016

[3] Toh SH, Coenen P, Howie EK, Straker LM. The associations of mobile touch screen device use with musculoskeletal symptoms and exposures: A systematic review. PLoS One. 2017;**12**(8):e0181220. DOI: 10.1371/journal.pone.0181220.

[4] American Optometric Association. Computer vision syndrome. 2021. Available from: https://www.aoa.org/healthy-eyes/eye-and-vision-conditions/computervision-syndrome? sso=y [Accessed: December 21, 2022]

[5] Ranasinghe P, Wathurapatha W, Perera Y, Lamabadusuriya D, Kulatunga S, Jayawardana N, et al. Computer vision syndrome among computer office workers in a developing country: An evaluation of prevalence and risk factors. BMC Research Notes. 2016;**9**(1):1-9. DOI: 10.1186/s13104-016-1962-1

[6] Mobile Consumer Survey: The Australian cut 2017: Deloitte. 2017. Available from: https://www2.deloitte.com/content/dam/Deloitte/au/Documents/technology-media-telecommunications/deloitte-au-tmt-mobile-consumer-survey-2017-211117-final.pdf. [Accessed: December 21, 2022]

[7] Eurofound. Sixth European Working Conditions Survey. 2017. Available from: https://www.eurofound.europa.eu/sites/default/files/ef_publication/field_ef_document/ef1634en.pdf [Accessed: December 21, 2022]

[8] De-Hita-Cantalejo C, Sánchez-González JM, Silva-Viguera C, Sánchez-González MC. Tweenager computer visual syndrome due to tablets and laptops during the Postlockdown COVID-19 pandemic and the influence on the binocular and accommodative system. Journal of Clinical Medicine. 2022;**11**(18):5317. DOI: 10.3390/jcm11185317

[9] Adane F, Alamneh YM, Desta M. Computer vision syndrome and predictors among computer users in Ethiopia: A systematic review and meta-analysis. Tropical Medicine and Health. 2022;**50**(1):26. DOI: 10.1186/s41182-022-00418-3

[10] Sheppard AL, Wolffsohn JS. Digital eye strain: Prevalence, measurement and amelioration. BMJ Open Ophthalmology. 2018;**3**(1):e000146. DOI: 10.1136/bmjophth-2018-000146

[11] Portello JK, Rosenfield M, Bababekova Y, Estrada JM, Leon A. Computer-related visual symptoms in office workers. Ophthalmic & Physiological Optics. 2012;**32**(5):375-382. DOI: 10.1111/j.1475-1313.2012.00925.x

[12] Al Tawil L, Aldokhayel S, Zeitouni L, Qadoumi T, Hussein S, Ahamed SS. Prevalence of self-reported computer vision syndrome symptoms and its associated factors among university students. European Journal of Ophthalmology. 2020;**30**(1):189-195. DOI: 10.1177/1120672118815110

[13] Iqbal M, Elzembely H, Elmassry A, Elgharieb M, Assaf A, Ibrahim O, et al. Computer vision syndrome prevalence and ocular sequelae among medical students: A university-wide study on a marginalized visual security issue. Open Ophthalmology Journal. 2021;**15**(1):156-170

[14] Gonzalez-Perez M, Susi R, Antona B, Barrio A, González E. The computer-vision symptom scale (CVSS17): Development and initial validation. Investigative Ophthalmology & Visual Science. 2014;**55**(7):4504-4511. DOI: 10.1167/iovs.13-13818

[15] Segui Mdel M, Cabrero-Garcia J, Crespo A, Verdú J, Ronda E. A reliable and valid questionnaire was developed to measure computer vision syndrome at the workplace. Journal of Clinical Epidemiology. 2015;**68**(6):662-673. DOI: 10.1016/j.jclinepi.2015.01.015

[16] Shahid E, Burhany T, Siddique WA, Fasih U, Shaikh A. Frequency of computer vision syndrome in computer users. Pakistan Journal of Ophthalmology. 2017;**33**:108-112

[17] Torrey J. Understanding computer vision syndrome. Employment Relations Today. 2003;**30**:45-51. DOI: 10.1002/ERT.10073

[18] Charpe NA, Kaushik V. Computer vision syndrome (CVS): Recognition and control in software professionals. Journal of Human Ecology. 2009;**28**(1):67-69. DOI: 10.1080/09709274.2009.11906219

[19] Blurry vision? Tear your eyes away from the computer. The Seattle Times. Available from: https://www.seattletimes.com/business/technology/tear-your-eyes-away-from-the-computer/ [Accessed: December 21, 2022]

[20] Das A, Shah S, Adhikari TB, Paudel BS, Sah SK, Das RK, et al. Computer vision syndrome, musculoskeletal, and stress-related problems among visual display terminal users in Nepal. PLoS One. 2022;**17**(7):e0268356. DOI: 10.1371/journal.pone.0268356

[21] Mohan A, Sen P, Shah C, Jain E, Jain S. Prevalence and risk factor assessment of digital eye strain among children using online e-learning during the COVID-19 pandemic: Digital eye strain among kids (DESK study-1). Indian Journal of Ophthalmology. 2021;**69**(1):140. DOI: 10.4103/ijo.IJO_2535_20

[22] Mohan Kumar B, Thiruvalluvan G, Arjunan M. Effectiveness on knowledge about computer vision syndrome among medical coding trainee in medical coding training institute in urban Chennai, Tamil Nadu – A cross- sectional study. Journal of Family Medicine and Primary Care. 2021;**10**(1):228. DOI: 10.4103/jfmpc.jfmpc_1151_20

[23] Natnael L, Dawit Z, Haile W, Anbesse D. Prevalence and associated factors of computer vision syndrome among bank workers in Gondar city, Northwest Ethiopia. Clinical Optometry. 2017;**9**:67-76. DOI: 10.2147/OPTO.S126366

[24] Seresirikachorn K, Thiamthat W, Sriyuttagrai W, Soonthornworasiri N, Singhanetr P, Yudtanahiran N, et al. Effects of digital devices and online learning on computer vision syndrome in students during the COVID-19 era: An online questionnaire study. BMJ Paediatrics Open. 2022;**6**(1):e001429. DOI: 10.1136/bmjpo-2022-001429

[25] Galindo-Romero C, Ruiz-Porras A, García-Ayuso D, Di Pierdomenico J, Sobrado-Calvo P, Valiente-Soriano FJ.

Computer vision syndrome in the spanish population during the COVID-19 lockdown. Optometry and Vision Science. 2021;**98**(11):1255-1262. DOI: 10.1097/OPX.0000000000001794

[26] Abusamak M, Jaber HM, Alrawashdeh HM. The effect of lockdown due to the COVID-19 pandemic on digital eye strain symptoms among the general population: A cross-sectional survey. Frontiers in Public Health. 2022;**10**:895517. DOI: 10.3389/fpubh.2022.895517

[27] Coronel-Ocampos J, Gómez J, Gómez A, Quiroga-Castañeda PP, Valladares-Garrido MJ. Computer visual syndrome in medical students from a private University in Paraguay: A survey study. Frontiers in Public Health. 2022;**10**:935405. DOI: 10.3389/fpubh.2022.935405

[28] Almalki AM, Alblowi M, Aldosari AM, Khandekar R, Al-Swailem SA. Population perceived eye strain due to digital devices usage during COVID-19 pandemic. International Ophthalmology. 2023:**43**(6):1935-1943. DOI: 10.1007/ s10792-022-02593-y

[29] Rosenfield M. Computer vision syndrome: A review of ocular causes and potential treatments. Ophthalmic & Physiological Optics. 2011;**31**(5):502-515. DOI: 10.1111/j.1475-1313.2011.00834.x

[30] Blehm C, Vishnu S, Khattak A, Mitra S, Yee RW. Computer vision syndrome: A review. Survey of Ophthalmology. 2005;**50**(3):253-262. DOI: 10.1016/j.survophthal.2005.02.008

[31] Alemayehu AM, Alemayehu MM. Pathophysiologic mechanisms of computer vision syndrome and its prevention: Review. World Journal of Ophthalmology & Vision Research. 2019;**2**(5):e1-e7. DOI: 10.33552/WJOVR.2019.02.00054

[32] Zhang D, Zhang WH, Dai SZ, Peng HY, Wang LY. Binocular vision and abnormal head posture in children when watching television. International Journal of Ophthalmology. 2016;**9**(5):746-749. DOI: 10.18240/ijo.2016.05.20

[33] Gur S, Ron S, Heicklen-Klein A. Objective evaluation of visual fatigue in VDU workers. Occupational Medicine (London). 1994;**44**(4):201-204. DOI: 10.1093/occmed/44.4.201

[34] Lee JW, Cho HG, Moon BY, Kim SY, Yu DS. Effects of prolonged continuous computer gaming on physical and ocular symptoms and binocular vision functions in young healthy individuals. Peer J. 2019;7:e7050. DOI: 10.7717/peerj.7050

[35] De-Hita-Cantalejo C, García-Pérez Á, Sánchez-González JM, Capote-Puente R, Sánchez-González MC. Accommodative and binocular disorders in preteens with computer vision syndrome: A cross-sectional study. Annals of the New York Academy of Sciences. 2021;**1492**:73-81

[36] Sheedy JE, Saladin JJ. Exophoria at near in presbyopia. American Journal of Optometry and Physiological Optics. 1975;**52**:474-481

[37] Tosha C, Borsting E, Ridder WH, Chase C. Accommodation response and visual discomfort. Ophthalmic & Physiological Optics. 2009;**29**(6):625-633. DOI: 10.1111/j.1475-1313.2009.00687.x

[38] Li R, Ying B, Qian Y, Chen D, Li X, Zhu H, et al. Prevalence of self-reported symptoms of computer vision syndrome and associated risk factors among school students in China during

the COVID-19 pandemic. Ophthalmic Epidemiology. 2022;**29**(4):363-373. DOI: 10.1080/09286586.2021.1963786

[39] Luberto F, Gobba F, Broglia A. Temporary myopia and subjective symptoms in video display terminal operators. La Medicina del Lavoro. 1989;**80**(2):155-163

[40] Altalhi A, Khayyat W, Khojah O, Alsalmi M, Almarzouki H. Computer vision syndrome among health sciences students in Saudi Arabia: Prevalence and risk factors. Cureus. 2020;**12**(2):e7060. DOI: 10.7759/cureus.7060

[41] Sánchez-Brau M, Domenech-Amigot B, Brocal-Fernández F, Quesada-Rico JA, Seguí-Crespo M. Prevalence of computer vision syndrome and its relationship with ergonomic and individual factors in Presbyopic VDT workers using progressive addition lenses. International Journal of Environmental Research and Public Health. 2020;**17**(3):1003. DOI: 10.3390/ijerph17031003

[42] Sánchez-Brau M, Domenech-Amigot B, Brocal-Fernández F, Seguí-Crespo M. Computer vision syndrome in presbyopic digital device workers and progressive lens design. Ophthalmic & Physiological Optics. 2021;**41**(4):922-931. DOI: 10.1111/opo.12832

[43] Kolbe O, Deble S. Presbyopic personal computer work: A comparison of progressive addition lenses for general purpose and personal computer work. Optometry and Vision Science. 2018;**95**(11):1046-1053. DOI: 10.1097/OPX.0000000000001295

[44] Logaraj M, Madhupriya V, Hegde S. Computer vision syndrome and associated factors among medical and engineering students in Chennai. Annals of Medical and Health Sciences Research. 2014;**4**(2):179-185. DOI: 10.4103/2141-9248.129028

[45] Kojima T, Ibrahim OM, Wakamatsu T, Tsuyama A, Ogawa J, Matsumoto Y, et al. The impact of contact lens wear and visual display terminal work on ocular surface and tear functions in office workers. American Journal of Ophthalmology. 2011;**152**(6):933-940.e2. DOI: 10.1016/j.ajo.2011.05.025

[46] Tauste A, Ronda E, Molina MJ, Segui M. Effect of contact lens use on computer vision syndrome. Ophthalmic & Physiological Optics. 2016;**36**(2):112-119. DOI: 10.1111/opo.12275

[47] Young G, Riley CM, Chalmers RL, Hunt C. Hydrogel lens comfort in challenging environments and the effect of refitting with silicone hydrogel lenses. Optometry and Vision Science. 2007;**84**(4):302-308. DOI: 10.1097/OPX.0b013e318042af0c

[48] Vertinsky T, Forster B. Prevalence of eye strain among radiologists: Influence of viewing variables on symptoms. AJR. American Journal of Roentgenology. 2005;**184**(2):681-686. DOI: 10.2214/ajr.184.2.01840681

[49] Himebaugh NL, Begley CG, Bradley A, Wilkinson JA. Blinking and tear break-up during four visual tasks. Optometry and Vision Science. 2009;**86**(2):106-114. DOI: 10.1097/OPX.0b013e318194e962

[50] Mowatt L, Gordon C, Santosh ABR, Jones T. Computer vision syndrome and ergonomic practices among undergraduate university students. International Journal of Clinical Practice. 2018;**72**(1):e13035. DOI: 10.1111/ijcp.13035

[51] Jainta S, Jaschinski W. Fixation disparity: Binocular vergence accuracy for a visual display at different positions relative to the eyes. Human Factors. 2002;**44**(3):443-450. DOI: 10.1518/0018720024497736

[52] Assefa NL, Weldemichael DZ, Alemu HW, Anbesse DH. Prevalence and associated factors of computer vision syndrome among bank workers in Gondar City, Northwest Ethiopia, 2015. Clinical Optometry. 2017;**9**:67-76. DOI: 10.2147/OPTO.S126366

[53] Agarwal S, Goel D, Sharma A. Evaluation of the factors which contribute to the ocular complaints in computer users. Journal of Clinical and Diagnostic Research. 2013;**7**(2):331-335. DOI: 10.7860/JCDR/2013/5150.2760

[54] Janosik E, Grzesik J. Influence of different lighting levels at workstations with video display terminals on operators' work efficiency. Medycyna Pracy. 2003;**54**(2):123-132

[55] Occupational Safety and Health Branch. LDahwlgh: A Guide to Work with Computers. 2010. Available from: https://www.labour.gov.hk/eng/public/oh/DisplayScreen.pdf. [Accessed: December 21, 2022]

[56] Larese Filon F, Drusian A, Ronchese F, Negro C. Video display operator complaints: A 10-year follow-up of visual fatigue and refractive disorders. International Journal of Environmental Research and Public Health. 2019;**16**(14):2501. DOI: 10.3390/ijerph16142501

[57] Tsubota K, Miyake M, Matsumoto Y, Shintani M. Visual protective sheet can increase blink rate while playing a hand-held video game. American Journal of Ophthalmology. 2002;**133**:704-705. DOI: 10.1016/s0002-9394(02)01389-2

[58] Calonge M, Pinto-Fraga J, Gonzalez-Garcia MJ, Enríquez-de-Salamanca A, López-de la Rosa A, Fernández I, et al. Effects of the external environment on dry eye disease. International Ophthalmology Clinics. 2017;**57**:23-40. DOI: 10.1097/IIO.0000000000000168

[59] Instituto Nacional de Seguridad y Salud en el Trabajo (INSST). Guía Técnica De Evaluación Y Prevención De Los Riesgos Relativos A La Utilización De Equipos Con Pantallas De Visualización. Madrid, Spain, 2021. Available from: https://www.insst.es/documents/94886/789467/Gu%C3%ADa+t%C3%A9cnica+para+la+evaluaci%C3%B3n+y+prevenci%C%B3n+de+los+riesgos+relativos+a+la+utilizaci%C3%B3n+de+equipos+con+pantallas+de+visualizaci%C3%B3n.pdf [Accessed: December 21, 2022]

[60] Zayed HAM, Saied SM, Younis EA, Atlam S. Digital eye strain: Prevalence and associated factors among information technology professionals, Egypt. Environmental Science and Pollution Research International. 2021;**28**(20):25187-25195. DOI: 10.1007/s11356-021-12454-3

[61] Long J, Cheung R, Duong S, Paynter R, Asper L. Viewing distance and eyestrain symptoms with prolonged viewing of smartphones. Clinical & Experimental Optometry. 2017;**100**(2):133-137. DOI: 10.1111/cxo.12453

[62] Altinbas E, Elibol A, Fıratlı G, Ayhan C, Celebi ARC. Assessment of risk factors on eye dryness in young adults using visual display device in both contact lens wearers and non-wearers. International Ophthalmology. 2022;**43**:1-10. DOI: 10.1007/s10792-022-02441-z

[63] Lemma MG, Beyene KG, Tiruneh MA. Computer vision syndrome

and associated factors among secretaries working in ministry offices in Addis Ababa, Ethiopia. Clinical Optometry. 2020;**12**:213-222. DOI: 10.2147/OPTO.S284934

[64] Maïssa C, Guillon M. Tear film dynamics and lipid layer characteristics—Effect of age and gender. Contact Lens Anterior Eye. 2010;**33**(4):176-182. DOI: 10.1016/j.clae.2010.02.003

[65] Dessie A, Adane F, Nega A, Wami SD, Chercos DH. Computer vision syndrome and associated factors among computer users in Debre Tabor town, Northwest Ethiopia. Journal of Environmental Public Health. 2018;**2018**:4107590. DOI: 10.1155/2018/4107590

[66] Ostrovsky A, Ribak J, Pereg A, Gaton D. Effects of job-related stress and burnout on asthenopia among high-tech workers. Ergonomics. 2012;**55**(8):854-862. DOI: 10.1080/00140139.2012.681808

[67] Sheedy JE, Hayes J, Engle J. Is all asthenopia the same? Optometry and Vision Science. 2003;**80**(11):732-739. DOI: 10.1097/00006324-200311000-00008

[68] Yang SN, Tai YC, Hayes JR, Doherty R, Corriveau P, Sheedy JE. Effects of font size and display quality on reading performance and visual discomfort of developmental readers. Optometry and Vision Science. 2010;**87**:E-abstract 105244

[69] Chu C, Rosenfield M, Portello JK, Benzoni JA, Collier JD. A comparison of symptoms after viewing text on a computer screen and paper. Ophthalmic & Physiological Optics. 2011;**31**(1):29-32. DOI: 10.1111/j.1475-1313.2010.00802.x

[70] Trusiewicz D, Niesluchowska M, Makszewska-Chetnik Z. Eye-strain symptoms after work with a computer screen. Klinika Oczna. 1995;**97**(11-12):343-345

[71] Shaw-McMinn PG. CVS: The practical and the clinical. Review of Optometry. 2001;**138**:78-88

[72] computer vision syndrome. Available from: https://www.aoa.org/healthy-eyes/eye-and-vision-conditions/computer-vision-syndrome?sso=y [Accessed: April 16, 2023]

[73] Lumoly V. Medical Practice and Review Impact of computer technology on health: Computer Vision Syndrome (CVS). Available from: https://www.academia.edu/28244623/Medical_Practice_and_Review_Impact_of_computer_technology_on_health_Computer_Vision_Syndrome_CVS [Accessed: December 21, 2022]

Chapter 4

Dry Eye and Allergic Conjunctivitis

Rachel Dandar and John Sheppard

Abstract

The primary goal of this chapter is to discuss the nuanced but prevalent clinical presentation of the patient with concurrent diagnoses of dry eye and allergic conjunctivitis. First, we discuss the epidemiology of dry eye disease and allergic conjunctivitis. We briefly discuss allergic blepharoconjunctivitis, a closely related entity with a different treatment focus. We thereafter discuss novel therapies, including loteprednol, varenicline nasal spray, reproxalap, and drug-eluting daily disposable soft contact lens. Lastly, we discuss a few biologic agents that hold promise for vernal and atopic keratoconjunctivitis, two forms of allergic eye disease that are more aggressive and can result in severe vision loss.

Keywords: tear film instability, ocular toxicity, allergic conjunctivitis, dry eye, allergic blepharoconjunctivitis

1. Introduction

Dry eye disease is a ubiquitous and often chronic condition, encountered frequently in ophthalmic practice. In 2017, more than 16 million Americans were afflicted by dry eye, approximately 6.8% of Americans [1]. Twice as common in women as in men, dry eye has also been demonstrated to increase in frequency with advancing age. With an aging population, the prevalence of dry eye will only increase. Typical symptoms of dry eye often include eye pain, grittiness, photophobia and blurred vision. The definition of dry eye disease was recently refined by the Tear Film & Ocular Surface Society International Dry Eye Workshop II (TFOS DEWS II) as "a multifactorial disease of the ocular surface characterized by a loss of homeostasis of the tear film, and accompanied by ocular symptoms, in which tear film instability and hyperosmolarity, ocular surface inflammation and damage, and neurosensory abnormalities play etiological roles" [2]. It should come as no surprise that additional ocular pathology, including meibomian gland dysfunction, allergic eye disease and iatrogenic factors, such as cataract surgery, can exacerbate dry eye by disrupting homeostasis of the tear film.

A variety of inflammatory ocular surface conditions can result in increased tear film osmolality and disruption of tear film homeostasis. Allergic conjunctivitis is classically associated with IgE-hypersensitivity to allergens. Within this cascade involves activation of mast cells, which results in an early response and a late phase response. The early response is associated with elevated levels of prostaglandins and histamine within the tear film [3]. The late response involves upregulation of interleukin-8 (IL-8) and macrophage inflammatory protein (MIP) [3]. Frequently, this presents clinically as tear film instability with inflamed conjunctival mucosa. In this chapter, we will focus on allergic eye disease as a concomitant diagnosis complicating the management of dry eye, in addition to highlighting novel treatments that are promising for the management of both conditions.

Allergy is a widespread condition, but ocular manifestations of allergic disease may be under-recognized within our current population. The first attempt at providing epidemiology on the incidence of specifically allergic eye disease was through data obtained between 1988 and 1994 [4]. While allergic rhinitis had previously been evaluated on prior censuses, allergic ocular symptoms had been overlooked. In this first evaluation, almost 30% of people had both nasal and ocular symptoms, with far fewer reporting ocular symptoms alone (6.4%). This study also revealed that isolated ocular symptoms are more common in patients as they age, typically over 50 years old, compared to combined nasal and ocular symptoms in younger age groups [4]. This should come as no surprise as it has already been thoroughly documented that the prevalence of atopy decreases with age whereas the prevalence of dry eye increases with age.

Like many diseases, allergic eye disease exists on a spectrum, with milder forms of allergy including seasonal allergic conjunctivitis (SAC) and perennial allergic conjunctivitis (PAC), ranging to the more severe atopic (AKC) or vernal keratoconjunctivitis (VKC). Whereas SAC and PAC classically impact the conjunctiva, VKC more frequently impacts the cornea and can severely reduce visual acuity through shield ulcers, vernal plaques and neovascularized scars [5]. As such, the treatments for allergic eye disease can vary widely in intensity depending on the severity of the presentation. VKC is more common among patients with concomitant atopic disease; as such, the more severe forms of ocular allergy are more likely to affect younger patients. Particularly for younger patients who may still be within the amblyogenic age range, aggressive management is indicated to combat corneal manifestations of VKC, in some cases requiring systemic therapies. For SAC and PAC, management is more often through topical therapies, but can become difficult when faced with coexistent dry eye.

In most studies related to ocular allergens, the predominant focus is most often on SAC and PAC as these are conditions more prevalent in older age groups, and thus within the work force. There are several well-documented allergens that are more likely to present with ocular symptoms as opposed to nasal symptoms: pet dander, dust, pollen, mold, and certain cosmetics. An additional interesting feature of this study was that the allergic disease was more prevalent in the southern United States, presumably secondary to higher humidity and relatively more pollen production [6]. With ongoing climate change and global warming, pollen production will continue to increase, suggesting that the prevalence of ocular allergy will only increase with time. Another consideration regarding ocular allergy prevalence includes the impact on vision, quality of life and economic productivity. While only 3% of adults have symptoms severe enough to prevent working outside of the home, the AIRS Survey revealed that the average self-reported decrease in productivity from allergic eye disease was 26 points, falling from a self-reported productivity of 91/100 with no allergic symptoms to 65/100 with the worst allergic symptoms [7]. As such, there is a need for effective therapies to mitigate the symptoms of allergic eye disease, to improve quality of life for those suffering from allergies and to enable these patients to continue to engage fully in their professions, instead of being limited by their symptoms.

Classic symptoms of allergic eye disease often overlap with those of dry eye, including redness, itching/pruritis, grittiness, burning, epiphora/tearing and blurred vision. However, allergic eye disease complicates the management of dry eye, as some treatments for stand-alone dry eye may not be as effective or as tolerable for the patient with concomitant allergic disease. Artificial tears may be considered as an initial therapy for patients with either dry eye or allergic conjunctivitis, but further treatment choices may become more difficult. It is not uncommon for muscarinic topical anti-histamines to dry the ocular surface, while topical therapies for dry eye and meibomitis frequently create hypersensitivity or irritative effects on the allergic ocular surface. Similarly, punctal plugs obviously would be a less desirable choice in a patient with allergic conjunctivitis, as this would result in prolonged exposure of the allergen to the ocular surface. Mast-cell stabilizers may be of utility in these patients, but can take days to weeks to reach peak efficacy, and as such, will not provide patients with immediate relief. As such, there is a need for more nuanced medications that can adequately address both allergic conjunctivitis and dry eye.

2. Allergic contact blepharoconjunctivitis

First, we will briefly discuss allergic contact blepharoconjunctivitis, a disease similar to SAC and PAC, but with slightly different management. The most common cause of an allergic contact blepharoconjunctivitis is the use of cosmetics. The inciting agent in these cases can include a variety of metal allergies, such as nickel, cobalt and chrome, as well as allergies to the fragrances added to these cosmetics [8]. While the solution for blepharoconjunctivitis in the setting of cosmetic use may be simple, allergen avoidance, it can often be difficult to pinpoint a cosmetic as the underlying cause of symptoms. Often, the history may be challenging. Women, who are twice as likely as men to experience symptoms of dry eye, are more likely to wear cosmetics, specifically mascara, on a daily basis. As such, their constellations of symptoms could easily be confused with an environmental allergen (akin to dust or dander). Furthermore, this allergic blepharoconjunctivitis may be exacerbated by the mechanical impact of cosmetic products. For example, application of mascara or eyeliner may obstruct meibomian gland orifices, which can lead to further team film instability and aggravation of dry eye and allergic symptoms [8]. As previously mentioned, dry eye is twice as common in women as in men, so providers must be aware of the impact of cosmetic use. For patients in whom allergen avoidance is less practical, such as those suffering from pollen allergies, there are a variety of novel therapies being released to attempt to better control the nuanced symptoms of concomitant dry eye and allergic eye disease.

3. Novel treatments for seasonal and perennial allergic conjunctivitis

One of the first efforts to address the inflammatory component of dry eye was the application of topical steroid therapy. In late 2020, KPI-121 0.25% (EYSUVIS, Kala Pharmaceuticals, Inc.) became the first commercially available mucus-penetrating particle (MPP) formulation of loteprednol etabonate ophthalmic emulsion approved for episodic dry eye. Investigated through the STRIDE trials, loteprednol etabonate was approved for four times daily (QID) use up to 2 weeks at a time [9, 10]. The mucus-penetrating particle vehicle enables the medication to avoid entrapment by conjunctival mucins and achieve better ocular penetration [9, 10]. For patients with a component of allergic disease, a low-dose topical steroid may be of particular use, as an intermittent topical steroid therapy may address underlying inflammation present in both dry eye and allergic disease. There are however some patients for whom a topical steroid may not be the best treatment option. For example, while there were no differences in intraocular pressure between the two STRIDE trial arms, loteprednol still has a higher rate of elevated intraocular pressure (IOP) than other topical medications such as olopatadine. As such, practitioners may still be hesitant to prescribe loteprednol for the patient with glaucoma, who may have a higher proclivity of IOP elevations [10]. Furthermore, as the medication is approved for only 2 weeks at a time, loteprednol would not be the best first choice for a patient with perennial symptoms.

Another medication that may be of particular interest for patients with both dry eye and allergy is Tyrvaya™ (varenicline solution) Nasal Spray. This novel dry eye treatment, initially approved in late 2021, enables a patient to avoid eye drops entirely. For some patients with either dry eye and/or allergic disease, application site reaction (i.e. burning pain on instillation of drops) may prohibit use of topical therapy. Tyrvaya™ could be considered in such patients, as the nasal spray circumvents this specific problem. Investigated by Ocean Point through the MYSTIC phase II randomized trial and the ONSET-2 Phase III Randomized Trial, Tyrvaya™ has repeatedly been shown to significantly improve signs and symptoms of dry eye [11, 12]. The primary endpoint in these studies was improvement in Schirmer's test by 10 mm or more by 4 out of 12 weeks of therapy; however, tear production was shown to increase as quickly as 5 minutes after administration [11]. While the exact mechanism of action is not completely understood, Tyrvaya™ is thought to be a neuro-stimulating agent, activating the parasympathetic pathway of the nasociliary branch of the trigeminal nerve in the nose, thereby increasing baseline tear production. Varenicline, the active ingredient in Tryvaya™, has previously been used as a smoking cessation aid. There is longstanding safety data for this medication, considering Chantix is used systemically in much higher doses with excellent tolerance. The side effect profile of Tyrvaya™ is relatively benign. The most common adverse reaction is sneezing, which occurs in 82% of patients. Cough, throat irritation and instillation-site (i.e. nose) irritation are among other common adverse reactions [11, 12].

While the use of Tryvaya™ in the setting of stand-alone allergic eye disease has not yet been investigated, for patients that suffer from both allergic eye disease and dry eye, Tryvaya™ may be of utility. Patients with a diagnosis of allergic rhinitis often use other medications administered via nasal spray to control their nasal symptoms, such as fluticasone, or FLONASE. For these patients, a nasal route of administration may be more-readily accepted, as they are familiar with/accustomed to this route of therapy. Given twice daily in each nostril, Tyrvaya™ can not only reduce topical treatment burden for patients, but is also an excellent option for patients who have difficulty with drops. Tyrvaya™ has advantages for patients with reduced neck mobility or reduced upper limb mobility, tremors, digital arthritis, patients who live alone and those who struggle self-administering eye drops. Another patient population that may benefit from Tyrvaya™ includes be the complex glaucoma patient who has developed allergic disease and toxicity in the form of medicamentosa. Of note, Tyrvaya™ has not been tested on patients with obstructive sleep apnea (OSA) who use continuous positive airway pressure (CPAP), with prior sinus surgeries, with a history of PKP, or those with recurrent nosebleeds [11]. As such, conclusions are unable to be drawn about its effectiveness in these specific demographics. Nevertheless, a single pharmaceutical with both a new delivery route and a novel mechanism of action holds great potential for patients afflicted by dry eye and allergic eye disease.

Another novel therapeutic, Reproxalap, is currently being investigated and developed by Aldyera to address both allergic conjunctivitis and dry eye disease. This topical medication is a novel, small-molecule immune-modulating covalent inhibitor of reactive aldehyde species (RASP) [13, 14]. While the exact mechanism of action of Reproxalap is not completely understood at this time, it is hypothesized to address the inflammatory component of both dry eye and allergic disease. RASP potentiate inflammation through a variety of inflammatory mediators and pathways, and as such, inhibition of RASP may inhibit the propagation of the inflammatory cascades.

Reproxalap was first evaluated in the treatment of dry eye alone in the Phase III TRANQUILITY trial. Participants were randomized to 0.1% reproxalap, 0.25% reproxalap and placebo groups. They were then exposed to a controlled adverse environment, consisting of low humidity for 90 minutes, after a 12-week course of QID treatment. Symptomatic relief was appreciated as early as 2 weeks into the treatment course, at the first follow up visit [13]. Patients experienced symptomatic improvement in a dose dependent response, particularly in relation to symptoms of grittiness and dryness [13]. Researchers also appreciated improvements in nasal fluorescein staining in the 0.25% group, so 0.25% Reproxalap QID was advanced to additional clinical trials. For patients with allergic conjunctivitis, Reproxalap was evaluated in a randomized, double-blind Phase IIb Trial and in the Phase III ALLEVIATE Trial [14, 15]. In each of these studies, participants were randomized to various treatment groups, including 0.25% Reproxalap, 0.5% Reproxalap and placebo. For both doses, participants who had been administered Reproxalap noted improvement in symptoms, notably tearing, itching and redness [14, 15]. However, participants taking the higher dose, 0.5% Reproxalap, experienced a higher rate of instillation site reaction, with higher rates of redness and irritation after the first dose, so the 0.25% regimen is being advanced [14]. Reproxalap is a promising medication for those suffering from both dry eye and allergic conjunctivitis.

Another novel therapeutic strategy currently under development are contact lenses impregnated and eluting a variety of different pharmaceutical agents. For patients who wear soft contact lenses, the current options for treatment of allergic conjunctivitis are limited. Topical drugs currently available, including ketotifen and olopatadine, are not recommended for use while soft contact lenses are in place due to the preservative benzalkonium chloride (BAK). For many patients, this translates to spectacle use during high allergy seasons in order to be able to instill anti-allergy drops and achieve symptomatic relief. There have been a variety of clinical trials in the past several years directed towards creation of drug-eluting daily disposable soft contact lens (DDSCL) [16]. The first DDSCL, Acuvue® Theravision™ with Ketotifen (ATK) (Johnson & Johnson Vision Care, Inc., Jacksonville, Florida, USA), was approved by the FDA in April of 2022. Prior to approval, multiple case studies were performed demonstrating subjective and objective improvement with use of ATK during high allergy seasons, with symptomatic relief of itch, and improvement in clinical features, including episcleral, ciliary and scleral injection, as well as extent of papillary reaction [17, 18]. It is thought that the ketotifen within the DDSCL is gradually released into lacrimal fluid below CL, to maintain therapeutic levels for longer, in contrast to topical drops, which have a more temporary effect as they are washed from the tear film.

A further consideration of a DDSCL as a therapeutic strategy is that a contact lens serves as a physical barrier, much like a bandage contact lens (BCL), in addition to the potential for a slow, sustained release of medication. As such, a DDSCL may be a parsimonious solution for a patient with both dry eye and ocular allergy. One current limitation of this specific therapy is that the toric options for DDSCL are currently limited to astigmatic errors of less than 1 diopter [16]. There have been additional studies regarding the creation of DDSCL with olopatadine and DDSCL with epinastine hydrochloride, but these have not yet entered human trials [19, 20]. Nonetheless, FDA approval of ATK as the first DDSCL is promising for the ophthalmic community, as ATK may enable patients to achieve better symptomatic control during high-allergy seasons, and DDSCL technology may expand to other ophthalmic conditions and enable patients to achieve better compliance with and tolerance of mediation regimens.

4. Novel treatments for atopic and vernal keratoconjunctivitis

Thus far we have focused primarily on novel therapies with a target audience of primarily patients who suffer from SAC and PAC. For patients afflicted by VKC, there have also been promising novel therapeutics developed over the last several years. While milder cases of VKC may be managed through topical and systemic anti-histamines, topical mast cell inhibitors, and tacrolimus ointment (0.03–0.1%), topical steroid dependence in these children is common and can result in a series of untoward side effects, including ocular hypertension, steroid-induced glaucoma and cataract. For children who are dependent on topical steroids, topical cyclosporine A (CsA, 0.5–2%) has been of great utility in partial or total reduction of topical steroid therapy. Unfortunately, topical CsA is ineffective for approximately 1/3 of children, and another 1/6 of children are still dependent on topical steroids despite topical CsA [21]. Omalizumab, a monoclonal, chimeric anti-IgE antibody has been used for allergic asthma since 1999 [22] and has recently garnered interest in the treatment of VKC. The underlying pathophysiology for the atopic triad, asthma, eczema and allergy, overlaps, with both IgE mediated and cell-mediated pathways provoking symptoms of the triad.

For patients with AKC and VKC, omalizumab has been used with some success. Delivered via subcutaneous injection, the dose and frequency of omalizumab therapy varied nearly fourfold among children, which may in part be related to the severity of the presentation and the extent of inflammatory levels in these patients [23]. Not all children had symptomatic improvement of ocular symptoms with omalizumab, which should come as no surprise, given approximately 50% of patients who suffer from VKC and/or AKC do not have an IgE-dependent immune response [24, 25]. For those children who experienced a response to omalizumab, often their symptoms of asthma and eczema improved as well [23].

Another consideration is that for some children, omalizumab alone was adequate to control symptoms, whereas for others, omalizumab alone did not adequately control symptoms. As such, there is a need for additional therapeutic targets for those with VKC and/or AKC arising through different mediators. Furthermore, omalizumab is not approved for the treatment of ocular allergy alone. Patients with severe symptoms would be best treated through multispecialty collaboration, with input from such specialties as Allergy, Immunology, Rheumatology, and/or Pulmonology for the prescription, dosing and management of these medications, as well as monitoring of the concomitant diseases. As such, omalizumab is a promising therapy for patients with severe VKC, and may help some, but not all, reduce their treatment burden.

For patients with AKC or VKC who have an incomplete or no response to omalizumab, another promising therapeutic target interleukin-5 (IL-5). IL-5 is a powerful, proinflammatory cytokine within the cell-mediated pathway of inflammation, affecting primarily eosinophils. Mepolizumab and reslizumab are humanized monoclonal antibodies that bind directly to IL-5, while benralizumab is anti-eosinophil monoclonal antibody that binds to the alpha subunit of the IL-5 receptor [26, 27]. Although none of these drugs have been studied in regards to allergic conjunctivitis, initial reports the treatment of patients with allergic and eosinophilic predominant asthma have been promising [28]. Given the common inflammatory cascades that result in the classic atopic triad, they may be considered potential future biologic therapies for patients with AKC and VKC.

5. Conclusions

Allergic eye disease, affecting around 1 in 3 Americans, is a ubiquitous condition and will likely only increase in prevalence as global warming and climate change result in higher temperatures and humidity. Existing on a wide spectrum, from milder forms like SAC and PAC, to more severe, vision-threatening forms in AKC and VKC, treatment of allergic eye disease can be complex, as it often coexists with dry eye disease. As novel medications with vastly different mechanisms of action and routes of administration are developed to address nuanced forms of dry eye and allergic disease, physicians will have more tools to address clinical signs and symptoms of dry eye and allergic eye disease in their patients.

Author details

Rachel Dandar[1*] and John Sheppard[1,2]

1 Department of Ophthalmology, Eastern Virginia Medical School, Norfolk, VA, USA

2 Virginia Eye Consultants/CVP Physicians, Norfolk, VA, USA

*Address all correspondence to: dandarr@evms.edu

References

[1] Farrand KF, Fridman M, Stillman IÖ, Schaumberg DA. Prevalence of diagnosed dry eye disease in the United States among adults aged 18 years and older. American Journal of Ophthalmology. 2017;**182**:90-98. DOI: 10.1016/j.ajo.2017.06.033

[2] Craig JP, Nichols KK, Akpek EK, et al. TFOS DEWS II definition and classification report. The Ocular Surface. 2017;**15**(3):276-283. DOI: 10.1016/j.jtos.2017.05.008

[3] La Rosa M, Lionetti E, Reibaldi M, et al. Allergic conjunctivitis: A comprehensive review of the literature. Italian Journal of Pediatrics. 2013;**39**:18. DOI: 10.1186/1824-7288-39-18

[4] Singh K, Axelrod S, Bielory L. The epidemiology of ocular and nasal allergy in the United States, 1988-1994. The Journal of Allergy and Clinical Immunology. 2010;**126**(4):778-783.e6. DOI: 10.1016/j.jaci.2010.06.050

[5] Villani E, Rabbiolo G, Nucci P. Ocular allergy as a risk factor for dry eye in adults and children. Current Opinion in Allergy and Clinical Immunology. 2018;**18**(5):398-403. DOI: 10.1097/ACI.0000000000000471

[6] Prince A, Norris MR, Bielory L. Seasonal ocular allergy and pollen counts. Current Opinion in Allergy and Clinical Immunology. 2018;**18**(5):387-392. DOI: 10.1097/ACI.0000000000000475

[7] Bielory L, Skoner DP, Blaiss MS, et al. Ocular and nasal allergy symptom burden in America: The allergies, immunotherapy, and rhinoconjunctivitiS (AIRS) surveys. Allergy and Asthma Proceedings. 2014;**35**(3):211-218. DOI: 10.2500/aap.2014.35.3750

[8] Norris MR, Bielory L. Cosmetics and ocular allergy. Current Opinion in Allergy and Clinical Immunology. 2018;**18**(5):404-410. DOI: 10.1097/ACI.0000000000000474

[9] Comstock TL, Sheppard JD. Loteprednol etabonate for inflammatory conditions of the anterior segment of the eye: Twenty years of clinical experience with a retrometabolically designed corticosteroid. Expert Opinion on Pharmacotherapy. 2018;**19**(4):337-353

[10] Venkateswaran N, Bian Y, Gupta PK. Practical guidance for the use of loteprednol etabonate ophthalmic suspension 0.25% in the management of dry eye disease. Clinical Ophthalmology. 2022;**16**:349-355

[11] Wirta D, Vollmer P, Paauw J, et al. Efficacy and safety of OC-01 (varenicline solution) nasal spray on signs and symptoms of dry eye disease: The ONSET-2 phase 3 randomized trial. Ophthalmology. 2021;**S0161-6420**(21):00836-00838. DOI: 10.1016/j.ophtha.2021.11.004

[12] Quiroz-Mercado H, Hernandez-Quintela E, Chiu KH, Henry E, Nau JA. A phase II randomized trial to evaluate the long-term (12-week) efficacy and safety of OC-01 (varenicline solution) nasal spray for dry eye disease: The MYSTIC study. The Ocular Surface. 2021;**24**:15-21. DOI: 10.1016/j.jtos.2021.12.007

[13] Clark D, Tauber J, Sheppard J, Brady TC. Early onset and broad activity of reproxalap in a randomized, double-masked, vehicle-controlled phase 2b trial in dry eye disease. American Journal of Ophthalmology. 2021;**226**:22-31. DOI: 10.1016/j.ajo.2021.01.011

[14] Clark D, Karpecki P, Salapatek AM, Sheppard JD, Brady TC. Reproxalap improves signs and symptoms of allergic conjunctivitis in an allergen chamber: A real-world model of allergen exposure. Clinical Ophthalmology. 2022;**16**:15-23. DOI: 10.2147/OPTH.S345324

[15] Clark D, Cavanagh B, Shields AL, Karpecki P, Sheppard J, Brady TC. Clinically relevant activity of the novel RASP inhibitor reproxalap in allergic conjunctivitis: The phase 3 ALLEVIATE trial. American Journal of Ophthalmology. 2021;**230**:60-67. DOI: 10.1016/j.ajo.2021.04.023

[16] Pall B, Gomes P, Yi F, Torkildsen G. Management of ocular allergy itch with an antihistamine-releasing contact lens. Cornea. 2019;**38**(6):713-717. DOI: 10.1097/ICO.0000000000001911

[17] A drug-eluting contact lens for allergic conjunctivitis. The Medical Letter on Drugs and Therapeutics. 2022;**18**:60-61. Available from: http://www.medicalletter.org/TML-article-1648c

[18] Ono J, Toshida H. Use of ketotifen fumarate-eluting daily disposable soft contact lens in management of ocular allergy: Literature review and report of two cases. Cureus. 2022;**14**(7):e27093. DOI: 10.7759/cureus.27093

[19] González-Chomón C, Silva M, Concheiro A, Alvarez-Lorenzo C. Biomimetic contact lenses eluting olopatadine for allergic conjunctivitis. Acta Biomaterialia. 2016;**41**:302-311. DOI: 10.1016/j.actbio.2016.05.032

[20] Minami T, Ishida W, Kishimoto T, et al. In vitro and in vivo performance of epinastine hydrochloride-releasing contact lenses. PLoS One. 2019;**14**(1):e0210362. DOI: 10.1371/journal.pone.0210362

[21] Doan S, Gabison E, Abitbol O, Gatinel D, Chast F, Hoang-Xuan T. Efficacy of topical 2% cyclosporine A as a steroid-sparing agent in steroid-dependent vernal keratoconjunctivitis. Journal Français d'Ophtalmologie. 2007;**30**(7):697-701. DOI: 10.1016/S0181-5512(07)91357-1

[22] Milgrom H, Fick RB Jr, Su JQ, Reimann JD, Bush RK, Watrous ML, et al. Treatment of allergic asthma with monoclonal anti-IgE antibody. rhuMAb-E25 study group. The New England Journal of Medicine. 1999;**341**(26):1966-1973. DOI: 10.1056/NEJM199912233412603

[23] Doan S, Amat F, Gabison E, Saf S, Cochereau I, Just J. Omalizumab in severe refractory vernal keratoconjunctivitis in children: Case series and review of the literature. Ophthalmology and Therapy. 2017;**6**(1):195-206. DOI: 10.1007/s40123-016-0074-2

[24] Bonini S, Bonini S, Lambiase A, Marchi S, Pasqualetti P, Zuccaro O, et al. Vernal keratoconjunctivitis revisited: A case series of 195 patients with long-term followup. Ophthalmology. 2000;**107**:1157-1163. DOI: 10.1016/S0161-6420(00)00092-0

[25] Bonini S, Coassin M, Aronni S, Lambiase A. Vernal keratoconjunctivitis. Eye. 2004;**18**:345-351. DOI: 10.1038/sj.eye.6700675

[26] Minami D, Kayatani H, Sato K, Fujiwara K, Shibayama T. Effectiveness of benralizumab for allergic and eosinophilic predominant asthma following negative initial results with omalizumab. Respirology Case Reports. 2018;**7**(1):e00388. DOI: 10.1002/rcr2.388

[27] Carpagnano GE, Pelaia C, D'Amato M, et al. Switching from omalizumab to mepolizumab:

Real-life experience from Southern Italy. Therapeutic Advances in Respiratory Disease. 2020;**14**:175346662092923. DOI: 10.1177/1753466620929231

[28] O'Reilly E, Casey D, Ibrahim H, et al. Real-world clinical outcomes in asthmatic patients switched from omalizumab to anti-interleukin-5 therapy. Journal of Asthma and Allergy. 2022;**15**:935-937. DOI: 10.2147/JAA.S358321

Section 3

Updates on Diagnosis

Chapter 5

Corneal Imaging Techniques for Dry Eye Disease

Robby Mattes, Marcela Huertas-Bello and Alfonso L. Sabater

Abstract

Dry eye disease (DED) is a common ocular disorder affecting millions worldwide. It is characterized by reduced tear production and/or increased tear evaporation, leading to ocular discomfort and impaired vision. Corneal imaging techniques are valuable tools for diagnosing and monitoring DED, as they can provide objective and quantitative information on the structure and function of the ocular surface and the tear film. This chapter will review the principles and applications of various corneal imaging techniques for DED, such as Slit-Lamp Biomicroscopy, Fluorescein CorneoGraphy, In Vivo Confocal Microscopy, Optical Coherence Tomography, Lipid Layer Interferometry, Topography, and Fluorophotometry. The advantages and limitations of each technique are discussed, as well as their potential role in future research and clinical practice, such as monitoring treatment efficacy and guiding personalized treatment approaches.

Keywords: corneal imaging, dry eye imaging biomarkers, dry eye disease, meibomian gland dysfunction, tear film evaluation

1. Introduction

DED is a widespread ocular ailment that impacts a significant number of individuals across the world. The condition is defined by a decrease in tear production, greater evaporation of tears, or changes in tear composition. Consequently, individuals may experience eye discomfort, vision abnormalities, and damage to the surface of their eyes. Corneal imaging methods are valuable resources for diagnosing and monitoring DED, as they can offer precise and quantifiable assessments of the structure and function of the cornea. Below we will elaborate on some of the most widely used corneal imaging techniques for DED in greater detail.

2. Slit-lamp biomicroscopy

Slit-lamp biomicroscopy (**Figure 1**) is a technique that allows the examination of the anterior and posterior segments of the eye using a high-intensity light source and a magnifying lens. It is a vital implement for diagnosing and managing various ocular conditions, such as DED, corneal injuries, corneal dystrophy, and cataracts.

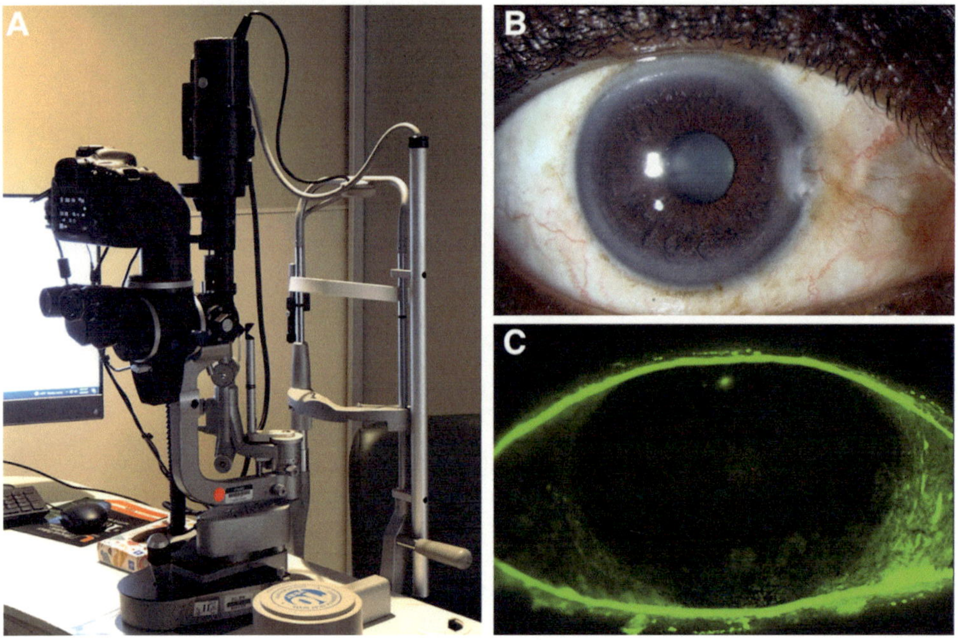

Figure 1.
(A) Slit-lamp biomicroscopy, a binocular microscope equipped with an adjustable light source, lenses for varying magnifications, and light filters. It allows examination of both the anterior and posterior segments of the eye, as well as performing diagnostic procedures. (B) Color photo of the anterior segment of the right eye in a patient with nasal pterygium, conjunctival melanosis, and gerontoxon. (C) Photo of the anterior segment of the eye with a cobalt-blue filter in a patient with fluorescein staining demonstrating superior and inferior corneal epithelial erosions.

2.1 Principles and applications

It consists of a binocular microscope and a light source that can be adjusted in width, height, angle, and intensity. The slit lamp can be combined with various accessories, such as lenses, filters, tonometers, and cameras, to perform additional diagnostic procedures [1]. This method can help to assess the severity of DED by measuring the tear film break-up time (TBUT), the tear meniscus height (TMH), and the presence of corneal and conjunctival staining as well as the underlying causes, such as meibomian gland dysfunction (MGD), blepharitis, or ocular surface inflammation [2].

Slit-lamp biomicroscopy is especially useful for studying contact lens wearers and DED patients who may have altered ocular surface microcirculation due to their conditions. It can reveal subtle changes in the blood flow and vessel density of the conjunctiva that may indicate the severity and progression of DED or the effects of contact lens wear [3].

2.2 Advantages and limitations

- It is noninvasive method.
- It can help in the early detection of DED.
- It provides high-resolution images of the ocular structures and microvasculature such as TMH.

- It allows the manipulation of illumination and magnification, facilitating the observation of different features of DED such as TBUT.

- It can help in monitoring disease progression.

While it is a valuable tool in the diagnosis of DED, it has some limitations that should be considered. Firstly, it is a subjective and qualitative method that relies heavily on the examiner's expertise and experience. Additionally, it may not provide a comprehensive understanding of the underlying causes, severity, or progression of DED. For instance, it cannot measure crucial indicators of DED such as tear osmolarity, tear production, tear evaporation rate, or inflammatory markers.

2.3 Potential role in future research and clinical practice

Researchers can use this technique to evaluate the accuracy and reliability of new diagnostic tools for DED, such as imaging technologies or tear film biomarkers. By comparing the results of these new tools with those obtained from traditional slit-lamp examinations, researchers can determine their usefulness in clinical practice. It can also be used to assess the effectiveness of treatments for DED, such as anti-inflammatory medications, artificial tears, and punctal occlusion. This technique allows them to measure changes in tear film quality, corneal staining, and other parameters, providing a reliable means of evaluating treatment efficacy for improving ocular surface health.

In clinical practice, it is used to assess the severity of corneal damage or DED by applying corneal grading scales. Some of the most commonly used corneal grading scales are the National Eye Institute/Industry Workshop (NEI) grading scale, the Oxford grading scale, and the Van Bijsterveld grading scale [4]. All three scales use a four-point grading system but differ in the number and location of regions evaluated, the type of dye used for the conjunctiva, and the illumination and magnification settings of the slit-lamp biomicroscopy [5].

This method can reveal signs of DED such as conjunctival hyperemia, corneal staining, tear film instability, and MGD [6]. Different filters can be used to enhance the visualization of these signs. For example, a cobalt-blue filter can be used with fluorescein dye to detect corneal epithelial defects or measure TBUT [7].

Overall, slit-lamp biomicroscopy is a valuable and versatile equipment in the diagnosis and management of DED, as well as other ocular conditions. Its ability to provide high magnification and illumination of the anterior and posterior segments of the eye allows for a detailed examination of its structures, function, and abnormalities. However, it should be used in conjunction with other diagnostic tools to accurately diagnose and manage DED. Furthermore, it has potential roles in future research to develop and evaluate new diagnostic tools and treatments for DED and investigate its underlying mechanisms.

3. In vivo confocal microscopy

In vivo confocal microscopy (IVCM) (**Figure 2**) is a noninvasive imaging technique that allows high-resolution and real-time visualization of cellular and subcellular structures of the cornea and other ocular tissues in living eyes. IVCM can provide information about the morphology, density, distribution, and function of various corneal structures, such as epithelial cells, immune cells, nerves, keratocytes, endothelial cells, and meibomian glands [8].

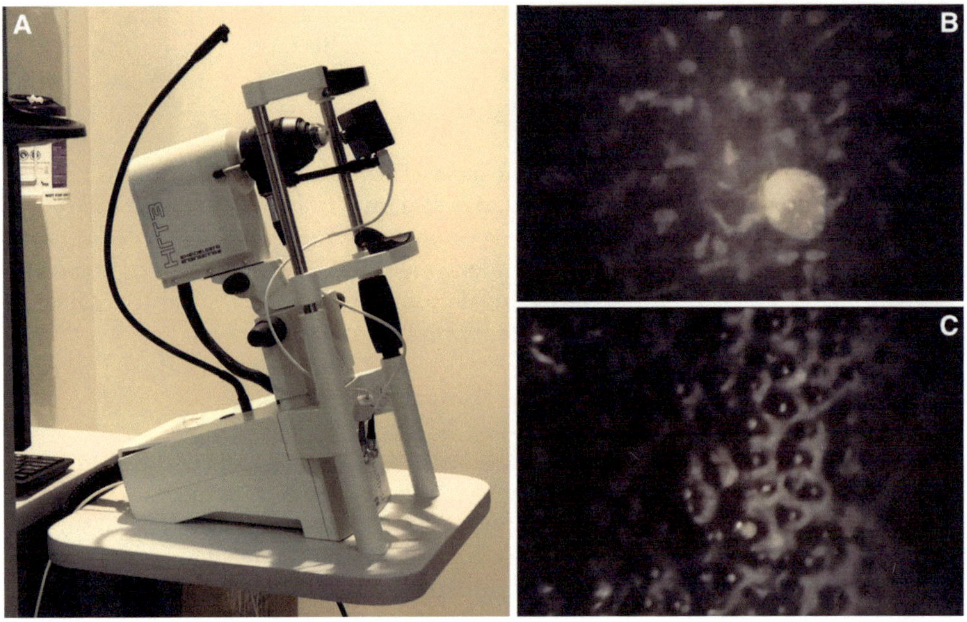

Figure 2.
(A) In vivo confocal microscopy is a noninvasive imaging technique that allows high-resolution, real-time visualization of cellular and subcellular ocular structures. (B) Corneal stromal opacities in a patient with fleck dystrophy. (C) Corneal endothelium with guttae in a patient with advanced Fuchs dystrophy.

3.1 Principles and applications

IVCM works by directing a laser beam onto a specific area, allowing for the detection of cellular structures through the reflection of light from a single focal plane [9]. By scanning different depths of tissue sequentially, it can generate high-resolution images that resemble histological sections. The microscope is able to capture these images of cells at different levels of depth, thus providing a noninvasive way to monitor changes in cells over time [8].

IVCM has various applications, such as studying corneal physiology and pathology, diagnosing infectious and inflammatory diseases, monitoring treatment efficacy, and guiding personalized treatment approaches [8, 10]. It can measure the density, morphology, branching pattern, tortuosity, reflectivity, length, and diameter of subbasal nerve plexus (SNP), which are altered in DED due to neurosensory abnormalities. SNP parameters can also correlate with clinical signs and symptoms of DED [11]. It can also quantify the density, size, shape, and activation state of dendritic cells (DCs), which are increased in DED due to inflammation. DCs parameters can also correlate with clinical signs and symptoms of DED [12]. IVCM can assess the morphology, density, and function of meibomian glands, which are impaired in evaporative dry eye (EDE) due to MGD. Meibomian gland parameters can also correlate with clinical signs and symptoms of EDE [13]. IVCM can diagnose DED more accurately by identifying specific features such as epithelial irregularity, microcysts, dendritic cells, nerve fiber loss, keratocyte activation, and meibomian gland dropout [8, 14]. Moreover, it can help monitor the progression of DED over time and evaluate the response to different treatments [15]. For example, it can show the effects of artificial tears on epithelial integrity, the effects of cyclosporine on inflammatory cell infiltration, or the effects of thermal pulsation therapy on meibomian gland function [16–18]. It can also assist in the diagnosis and management of corneal and conjunctival diseases, as well as the monitoring of postsurgical outcomes [19–21].

3.2 Advantages and limitations

It has several advantages over conventional histology because of its noninvasive nature, such as providing real-time images without tissue processing or staining, eliminating the need for tissue biopsy, reducing the risk of infection and scarring. It can detect subtle changes in the ocular surface that may not be visible with slit-lamp examination or staining techniques. For example, it can reveal epithelial cell loss, microcysts, basal cell density reduction, keratocyte activation, nerve fiber alterations, inflammatory cell infiltration, vascularization, and fibrosis in DED patients [8, 22]. IVCM can quantify these changes using objective parameters such as cell density, cell size, cell shape index, nerve fiber length, nerve fiber density, nerve branch density, nerve tortuosity, meibomian gland acinar unit density, meibomian gland acinar unit diameter, meibomian gland fibrosis grade, etc., which can help monitor disease progression and treatment response [20, 23]. It can also differentiate between different types and subtypes of DED based on their distinct ocular surface features. For example, it can help distinguish between the aqueous-deficient dry eye (ADDE) and EDE, as well as between obstructive MGD and nonobstructive MGD [24].

IVCM also allows for repeated imaging with quantitative analysis of morphological parameters making it an excellent tool for monitoring treatment efficacy and disease progression. Additionally, it can be used to assess eye conditions at the cellular level, providing detailed information on disease mechanisms and aiding in developing personalized treatment approaches.

However, it has some limitations, such as limited penetration depth, variability in image quality and interpretation, lack of standardized protocols and criteria for diagnosis, and potential risks of corneal damage or infection from contact probes [8]. It has a small field of view (~400×400 micrometers), which may not represent the whole ocular surface area or capture regional variations. Therefore, multiple images from different locations are needed to obtain a comprehensive assessment [25]. It also lacks population-based norms or standardized criteria for normal or abnormal findings.

Therefore, the interpretation and quantification of IVCM images may vary depending on the operator's experience or software used. Moreover, the correlation between IVCM parameters and clinical symptoms or signs is not always consistent or linear. It is still an expensive and relatively rare device that is not widely available or accessible, limiting its use in clinical practice [26].

3.3 Potential role in future research and clinical practice

The diagnosis and management of DED can be challenging, as no single test can reliably assess the severity and etiology of the condition [27]. Furthermore, there may be a discrepancy between clinical signs and symptoms of DED, as some patients may have significant ocular surface damage without experiencing discomfort, while others may report severe discomfort with minimal signs [28].

The following findings suggest that IVCM is an important tool that has a potential role in future research and clinical practice of DED, as it can provide valuable insights into the pathophysiology, diagnosis, classification, and treatment response of its different subtypes:

- It has been shown that patients with ADDE have reduced density and increased tortuosity of corneal subbasal nerves compared to healthy controls, while patients with EDE have increased density and decreased tortuosity of these nerves compared to ADDE patients [24].
- It has also shown that patients with MGD have altered morphology and function of meibomian glands compared to healthy controls, such as decreased acinar density, increased acinar size variability, increased ductal dilation, etc. These changes correlate with clinical signs such as meibum quality, meibum expressibility, etc. [29].
- It has demonstrated that various treatments for DED can improve ocular surface parameters such as corneal epithelial cell density, corneal nerve density and morphology, meibomian gland morphology and function, etc. [30].
- It can be used to evaluate the corneal and conjunctival epithelium, monitor graft survival after transplantation, and evaluate the effectiveness of topical medications [31].

In summary, IVCM is a noninvasive imaging technique that allows for the visualization of living cells and tissues in situ. Although it has limitations, it can provide detailed cellular information that boosts our understanding of ocular surface diseases and improves eye care management for further research and clinical practice [32].

4. Optical coherence tomography

Optical coherence tomography (OCT) (**Figure 3**) is a noninvasive imaging technique that uses low-coherence light to capture micrometer-resolution, two- and

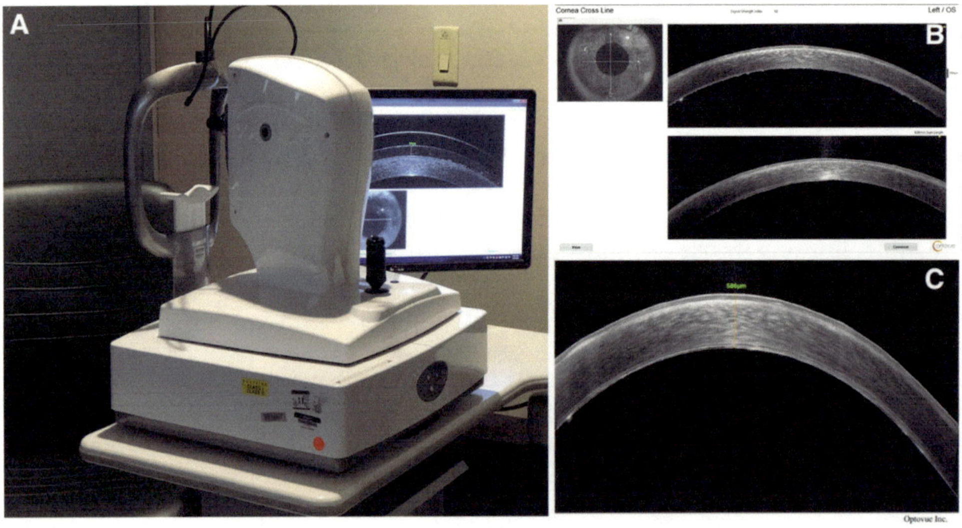

Figure 3.
(A) Optical coherence tomography is a noninvasive imaging technique that uses low-coherence light to capture micron-resolution two- and three-dimensional images creating high-resolution images of biological tissues. (B) Anterior segment optical coherence tomography in a healthy patient. (C) Pachymetry module (corneal thickness).

three-dimensional images creating high-resolution images of biological tissues. It is effectively 'optical ultrasound', imaging reflections from within tissue to provide cross-sectional images. OCT has become vital equipment in medical diagnosis and research due to its ability to provide detailed information about tissue microstructure and function. It is widely used for medical imaging and industrial nondestructive testing (NDT).

4.1 Principles and applications

OCT is based on the principle of low-coherence interferometry, which measures the interference pattern of two coherent light beams. The wavelength used is around 1300 nm to minimize energy absorption in the light beam caused by protein, water, hemoglobin, and lipids. The physics principle that allows the filtering of scattered light is optical coherence [33, 34].

It exploits the fact that coherent light can be split into two beams by a beam splitter: one beam (the reference beam) travels along a known path length and reflects off a mirror, while the other beam (the sample beam) travels through the tissue of interest and reflects off various structures within it [35]. The two beams are then recombined by another beam splitter and detected by a photodetector [36]. The interference pattern produced by the recombined beams depends on the difference in optical path length between them [37]. By varying the position of the reference mirror, different depths within the tissue can be scanned and imaged [38].

There are different types of OCT systems based on how they vary the reference path length and how they detect the interference signal. The most common types are time-domain OCT (TD-OCT), frequency-domain OCT (FD-OCT), and swept-source OCT (SS-OCT) [38, 39].

- TD-OCT uses a moving reference mirror to scan different depths within the tissue sequentially. The interference signal is detected as a function of time by a single photodetector [40].

- FD-OCT uses a fixed reference mirror and measures the interference signal as a function of wavelength by using an array of photodetectors or a spectrometer. This allows simultaneous acquisition of all depths within the tissue without mechanical scanning [41].

- SS-OCT uses a tunable laser source that sweeps across different wavelengths rapidly. The interference signal is detected as a function of time by a single photodetector synchronized with the laser sweep [42].

FD-OCT and SS-OCT offer higher speed, sensitivity, and resolution than TD-OCT because they avoid mechanical scanning and use more efficient detection methods [43].

OCT has many applications in biomedical imaging due to its ability to provide high-resolution cross-sectional images of tissue microstructure without requiring invasive procedures or contrast agents [38]. It can provide valuable information about the corneal epithelial thickness (CET), which reflects the health and integrity of the ocular surface [44]. In addition, OCT can image different layers of the cornea, anterior and posterior chamber, etc., providing valuable information for diagnosing and monitoring diseases such as keratoconus, corneal disorders, glaucoma, diabetic retinopathy, age-related macular degeneration, etc. [45].

4.2 Advantages and limitations

One of the primary advantages is its noninvasive nature, which allows for repeat imaging of tissues. Additionally, OCT can provide real-time imaging, which can aid in surgical procedures, reducing the chances of error because it is a computerized procedure [46]. It has several advantages over other imaging modalities; some of these advantages are:

- High resolution: it can achieve submicrometer axial resolution and micrometer lateral resolution in tissue, which allows visualization of cellular-level features that are not accessible by other techniques [47].

- High speed: it can acquire images at rates up to hundreds of frames per second or even megahertz range with FD-OCT methods, which enables real-time feedback during interventions or dynamic studies [38].

- Noninvasiveness: it does not require ionizing radiation or contrast agents that may pose health risks or cause allergic reactions. It also does not require physical contact with the sample except for intravascular applications [48].

- Versatility: it can be integrated with various endoscopic devices or surgical instruments to enable minimally invasive imaging in different anatomical locations, for example, some devices can combine OCT with other modalities like confocal scanning laser ophthalmoscopy (cSLO) or indocyanine green angiography (ICG) [49].

However, it also has some limitations; for instance, it may not capture subtle changes in CET that occur in the mild or early stages of DED. Moreover, OCT measurements of CET may vary depending on the device type, scanning protocol, calibration method, and image processing algorithm [50].

Some other limitations are:

- It is expensive and not always covered by insurance.

- It requires patient cooperation and operator skill.

- It may produce image artifacts and distortions due to eye movements, blinking, or scanning errors.

- It is sensitive to tissue optical properties, and tissues with different optical properties may not be imaged with the same resolution.

- It has a limited penetration depth due to multiple scattering effects within tissue, and OCT typically has a penetration depth ranging from 1 to 3 mm depending on tissue type, which restricts its ability to image deeper tissues [45, 51, 52].

4.3 Potential role in future research and clinical practice

Recently, OCT has also shown potential for diagnosing and managing DED [53]. It can measure parameters such as TMH, CET, and meibomian gland morphology, which are related to DED severity and symptoms. By integrating OCT-derived data into a new scoring method, researchers have proposed a more objective and accurate way of assessing DED [54]. Therefore, it may play an important role in future DED research and clinical practice by providing novel insights into its pathophysiology, diagnosis, and treatment [55].

One area where OCT is being used is in monitoring treatment efficacy [56]. For example, it can be used to monitor changes in tissue microstructure and function following treatment for diseases such as cancer, and it can also be used to measure retinal nerve fiber layer thickness, macular thickness, choroidal thickness, optic nerve head parameters, etc., which can reflect the progression or regression of various eye diseases [57, 58]. Additionally, it can be used to guide personalized treatment approaches by providing information about tissue structure and function [59].

Another area where it has potential is developing new imaging agents. Researchers are exploring using OCT in combination with contrast agents to improve image contrast and sensitivity, which could allow for earlier detection of diseases [60].

In conclusion, OCT is a very resourceful method with various clinical and research applications. While it has some limitations, its noninvasive nature and high-resolution images make it an attractive option for diagnosing and monitoring eye diseases such as DED.

5. Lipid layer interferometry

Lipid layer interferometry (LLI) (**Figure 4**) is a technique that uses light interference patterns to measure the thickness, stability, and quality of the lipid layer in vivo. LLI is a promising tool for diagnosing and managing DED caused by MGD. It can provide objective and quantitative information about the lipid layer quality and guide treatment decisions based on individual patient needs.

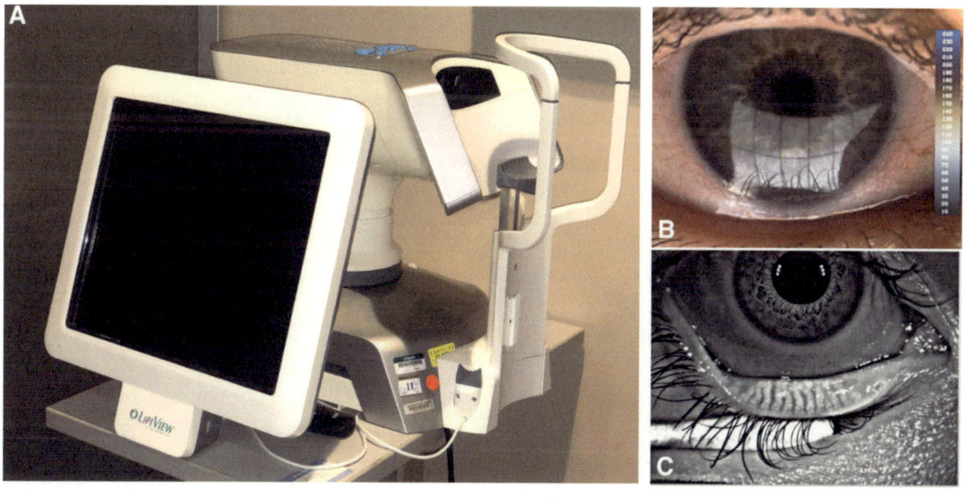

Figure 4.
(A) Lipid layer interferometry is a technique that uses light interference patterns to measure the thickness, stability, and quality of the lipid layer in vivo. (B) Tear film image. (C) Meibomian gland imaging in a patient with dry eye syndrome.

5.1 Principles and applications

LLI works by shining a beam of polarized light onto the tear film and capturing the reflected light with a camera—the reflected light forms an interference pattern that depends on the thickness and uniformity of the lipid layer. The interference pattern can be analyzed using software algorithms to calculate the lipid layer thickness (LLT) in nanometers (nm) or interferometric color units (ICU), which are close but not exactly equivalent to nm, and classify their appearance into different grades [61]. A normal LLT ranges from 80 to 120 nm (or ICU), while a thin LLT is below 60 nm (or ICU). A thick LLT above 100 nm (or ICU) may indicate excessive meibum production or altered tear film dynamics [42]. Different thicknesses produce different colors according to a specific scale. For example, white indicates a very thin LLT (<20 nm), while yellow indicates a thick LLT (>100 nm) [62].

LLI can provide quantitative and qualitative information about the lipid layer in DED patients, which can help diagnose and monitor their condition [61]. The lipid layer prevents excessive evaporation of tears and provides lubrication for blinking [63].

One of the devices that use LLI is LipiView II (Johnson & Johnson Vision), which measures the LLT between blinks and gives a numerical value in ICU units close to nanometers [64]. LipiView II also captures images of the lipid layer spread (LLS), which reflects how well the lipid layer covers and smooths out after each blink. A normal LLS is considered to be uniform and continuous [64, 65]. Several studies have shown that LLI can be useful for assessing DED severity and treatment response. For example, a study by Yunji Lee Et al. found that DED patients had significantly lower LLT and LLS than healthy controls and that LLT correlated with TBUT and ocular surface staining scores. They also found that DED patients with thick LLT (>100 ICU) had different characteristics than those with thin LLT (<100 ICU), such as higher TBUT, lower osmolarity, and lower inflammatory markers [66].

5.2 Advantages and limitations

LLI provides a noninvasive, real-time, and quantitative measurement of the thickness and quality of the lipid layer, enabling the study of various interventions effects on it and ocular surface health [67, 68]. LLI has also been shown to have good reproducibility and sensitivity in detecting changes in the lipid layer [68]. Additionally, LLI has been used to evaluate DED and MGD [69–72].

In summary:

- Noninvasive and real-time method for quantitatively measuring the thickness and quality of the lipid layer in the tear film.
- Good reproducibility and sensitivity in detecting changes in the lipid layer.
- Enables the study of various interventions' effects on the lipid layer and ocular surface health.
- Useful for evaluating DED, contact lens wear, and meibomian gland dysfunction.

- Noninvasive and does not require contact with the eye or the instillation of any dye or drops.
- Provides quantitative and objective measurements of LLT that can be compared over time or between groups.
- Can detect subtle changes in LLT that may not be visible with other techniques.
- Reveals spatial variations in LLT across different regions of the eye.

However, it also has some limitations and challenges:

- The technique may have a limited ability to discriminate between thin lipid layers, as measurements may be affected by the instrument's sensitivity and resolution [71]. Secondly, LLI may not provide a complete picture of the lipid layer structure, as it only provides measurements of the LLT and quality, not its composition or structure [73].
- Some researchers have suggested that LLI measurements may be influenced by environmental factors such as temperature and humidity, which may affect the behavior of the lipid layer [74, 75].
- Finally, LLI measurements may be affected by the ocular surface curvature, refractive errors, blinking artifacts, or variations in the tear film during the measurement process [71].

5.3 Potential role in future research and clinical practice

One potential application is the evaluation of therapeutic interventions, such as topical lipid-based treatments, in improving the LLT and quality. Studies have shown that LLI can detect subtle changes in the lipid layer that may not be visible with other techniques, making it a useful tool in the assessment of DED [76]. In addition, the use of LLI may help in the identification of patients who are more likely to benefit from certain treatments, as well as to monitor the response to therapy [77].

Another potential application is in the assessment of MGD. Studies have shown a correlation between MGD severity and the quality of the lipid layer [78]. LLI may therefore be useful in the diagnosis and monitoring of MGD and in evaluating the effectiveness of treatments targeted at improving meibomian gland function [79]. LLI has been used to evaluate the effects of contact lenses on the LLT and quality [80]. In addition, it may be useful in the assessment of contact lens materials and designs and in developing new contact lens solutions aimed at improving the lipid layer and reducing symptoms of dryness and discomfort [81].

In conclusion, LLI is a promising tool for diagnosing and managing DED caused by MGD. It provides a noninvasive, real-time, and quantitative measurement of the thickness and quality of the lipid layer. LLI has been shown to have good reproducibility and sensitivity in detecting changes in the lipid layer, making it a valuable tool for understanding its role in the tear film and its impact on ocular surface health. However, LLI has some limitations and challenges and should be used in conjunction with other diagnostic methods to obtain a comprehensive evaluation of DED etiology and severity.

6. Topography

Topography (**Figure 5**) is a corneal imaging technique that provides detailed 3D maps of the cornea's shape and curvature. It detects corneal diseases and irregular corneal conditions, such as swelling, scarring, abrasions, deformities, and irregular astigmatisms [82]. It can also monitor the progression of DED and co-existing eye diseases, such as pterygium. It is an essential tool for refractive surgery candidates with DED, as it can measure CET and assess suitability for surgery [83].

6.1 Principles and applications

Corneal topography uses three principles: Placido disc reflection, Scanning slit technology, or Scheimpflug photography. It works by projecting a luminous object onto the cornea and analyzing its reflection.

There are different methods of corneal topography, such as the Placido method, slit scanning technique, and Schiempflug method [84–86]. The Placido method uses concentric rings of light to create a pattern on the cornea that can be captured by a camera [87]. The slit scanning technique uses a rotating slit beam to scan the cornea at different depths [86]. The Schiempflug method uses a rotating camera and light source that are tilted at an angle to capture images of both the anterior and posterior surfaces of the cornea [86]. Corneal topography can provide valuable information about the quality of vision and guide surgical planning for procedures such as laser refractive surgery, cataract surgery, and corneal transplantation [85]. This method can provide useful information for diagnosing and monitoring corneal diseases, planning refractive surgery, fitting contact lenses, evaluating postoperative outcomes, etc. It can be used to characterize the shape of the cornea, specifically, the anterior

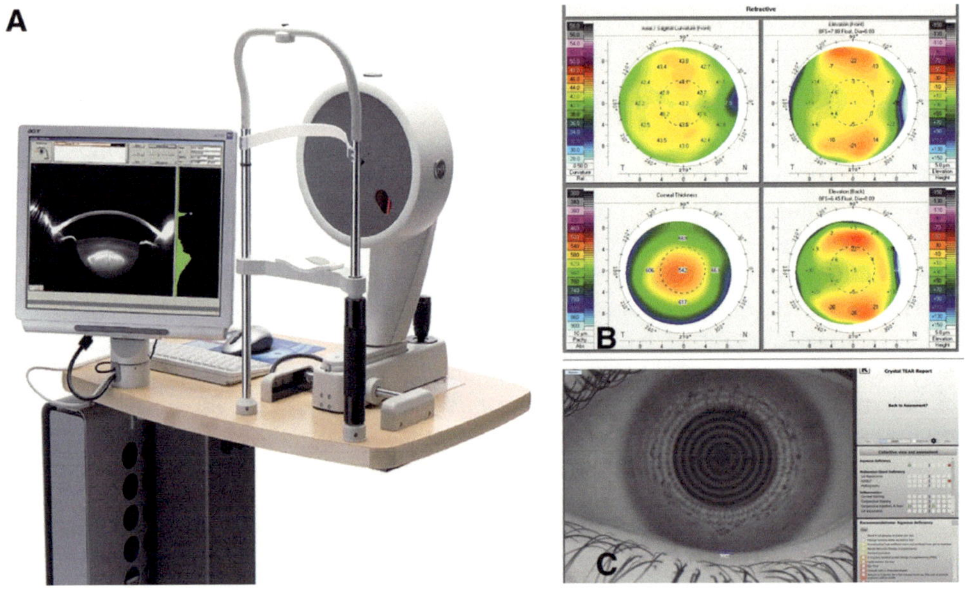

Figure 5.
(A) Corneal topography is an imaging technique of the cornea that provides detailed 3D maps of the shape and curvature of the cornea. (B) Corneal topography in a patient with mild corneal astigmatism. (C) Placido ring illumination and measurement of the tear meniscus.

surface of the cornea. Most corneal topographical systems are based on Placido discs that analyze rings that are reflected off the corneal surface [88]. The posterior corneal surface cannot be characterized using Placido disc technology [88].

Corneal topography is a technique that is also used to measure the thickness of the cornea [89]. It has been used to assess the effect of dry eye treatment on corneal thickness. Precise corneal topography measurements are essential for co-existing eye diseases in DED (DED) patients [90]. The tear film instability and hyper-osmolarity, ocular surface inflammation and damage, and neuro-sensory abnormalities play etiological roles [90]. Studies have been conducted to assess the repeatability of corneal topography measurements in dry eye patients and healthy controls [90, 91].

6.2 Advantages and limitations

- It can detect subtle changes in the corneal surface that may indicate DED, such as swelling, scarring, abrasions, or deformities. These changes can affect vision quality and increase the risk of infection or inflammation [88].

- It can help monitor the progression and severity of DED by measuring parameters such as corneal thickness, curvature, astigmatism, and irregularity. These parameters can reflect the degree of damage to the cornea caused by DED and guide treatment decisions [88, 92, 93].

- It can help evaluate the effectiveness of treatments for DED by showing improvements or worsening in corneal parameters after interventions such as artificial tears, punctal plugs, cyclosporine drops, or surgery.

However, it has some limitations when it comes to assessing DED. Here are some of them:

- It is unable to directly evaluate the quality or quantity of the tear film. Its findings only indicate the effect of DED on the cornea, which means it may not detect mild or early stages of DED that have not yet resulted in significant corneal changes [94].

- It may be influenced by factors other than DED, such as contact lens wear, ocular surgery, allergies, or infections. These factors may cause false-positive or false-negative results when evaluating DED with corneal topography [95].

- It may not be consistent or repeatable in severe cases of DED.

- It may not be covered by insurance for DED diagnosis.

6.3 Potential role in future research and clinical practice

- Developing new algorithms and models to improve the accuracy and reliability of corneal measurements [96, 97].

- Exploring novel parameters and indices to better characterize corneal shape and biomechanics.

- Investigating correlations between corneal topography and other ocular or systemic factors, such as intraocular pressure, tear film quality, diabetes mellitus, etc.

- Evaluating outcomes and complications of emerging surgical techniques or devices that modify corneal shape or function.

- Comparing different modalities or brands of corneal topography devices to establish standards and norms.

- A study found that corneal topography measurements could be used to predict corneal strength and resistance to deformation [98]. These findings suggest that corneal topography may have a valuable role in evaluating ocular biomechanics, which could be useful in diagnosing and monitoring various eye diseases.

It can be useful for several purposes in the clinical practice of DED:

- Screening: It can help identify patients who may have DED or are at risk of developing it by showing signs of irregularity or distortion in the corneal surface. For example, patients with MGD may show increased central corneal steepening due to tear film instability. Patients with Sjögren syndrome (SS) may show decreased central corneal thickness due to chronic inflammation [90].

- Diagnosis: It can help confirm or rule out DED by showing objective evidence of ocular surface damage or alteration due to tear film dysfunction. For example, patients with DED may show reduced TBUT. It can also measure TBUT by capturing images of the cornea at different intervals after blinking and calculating how long it takes for irregularities to appear [95]. Patients with DED may also show increased staining of the cornea with fluorescein dye due to epithelial defects or erosions. It can quantify staining by analyzing the intensity and distribution of fluorescence on the cornea.

- Monitoring: It can help track the progression or improvement of DED by showing changes in the corneal surface over time.

- It can measure CII by comparing different regions of the cornea and calculating how much they deviate from an ideal spherical shape [88, 99]. Patients with DED may also show worsening or improvement in their ocular surface disease index (OSDI). It may correlate OSDI scores with objective parameters such as TBUT, staining, and CII [100].

In conclusion, corneal topography is a valuable diagnostic and treatment tool for various ocular conditions such as DED. It also provides opportunities for advancing knowledge and innovation in ophthalmology. However, alone it is insufficient for diagnosing or treating DED. It must be used in conjunction with other tests and methods, including patient history, symptom assessment, tear film evaluation (e.g., Schirmer test), ocular surface staining (e.g., fluorescein), meibomian gland function (e.g., meibography), and inflammatory markers (e.g., MMP-9).

7. Fluorophotometry

Fluorophotometry is a technique that uses a device called a fluorophotometer to measure the fluorescence intensity of a dye called fluorescein after it is applied to the eye. Fluorescein is a yellow-green dye that binds to damaged cells on the corneal surface and emits light when exposed to blue light. It can provide information about various aspects of DED, such as corneal epithelial integrity and permeability, by measuring how much fluorescein penetrates into the cornea and how fast it is eliminated from the eye. It can also yield data concerning tear film stability, tear turnover rate and aqueous humor flow rate [101].

7.1 Principles and applications

It is based on the principle that some molecules (fluorophores) can absorb light at a certain wavelength (excitation) and emit light at a longer wavelength (emission). The intensity of the emitted light depends on several factors, such as the concentration of the fluorophore, the optical properties of the tissue, and the presence of quenchers or enhancers.

Fluorescein is a commonly used fluorophore for ocular fluorometry because it has a high quantum yield (the ratio of photons emitted to photons absorbed), low toxicity, and good solubility in water. Fluorescein has an excitation peak at 490 nm (blue light) and an emission peak at 520 nm (green light) [102].

To perform this technique, a known amount of fluorescein solution is instilled into the eye using a calibrated micropipette or strip. After allowing some time for diffusion and clearance of excess dye from the ocular surface, a fluorometer device is used to scan different regions of interest within the eye [103]. The fluorometer consists of an excitation source (usually a xenon arc lamp), an optical system (including filters or monochromators), a photodetector (usually a photomultiplier tube), and an electronic system for data acquisition and analysis [104]. The fluorometer measures the fluorescence intensity at each point along a scan line across the eye. The fluorescence intensity can be converted into concentration units using calibration curves obtained from standard solutions [105]. The concentration profiles can then be plotted as functions of location within the eye or time after dye instillation.

This method can be used to evaluate several parameters related to DED:

- Corneal epithelial permeability: It can measure this parameter by calculating the rate or extent of fluorescein penetration across the cornea [106]. This can reflect the degree of epithelial injury or dysfunction in DED patients.

- Tear film stability: It can measure this parameter by calculating the decay rate or half-life of fluorescein concentration on the corneal surface [103]. This can reflect the quality and stability of the tear film in DED patients.

- Tear turnover rate: This can reflect tear production and drainage imbalances, which may contribute to ocular surface irritation and inflammation in DED patients [106, 107].

7.2 Advantages and limitations

- It is objective and quantitative: it provides numerical values that can be compared across different individuals or time points [103].

- It is noninvasive: it does not require any contact with the eye surface or any tissue sampling [103].
- It is sensitive: it can detect subtle changes in the corneal epithelium that may not be visible with other methods such as slit-lamp examination or staining [103].
- It is specific: it measures only the permeability of the corneal epithelium, which is directly related to its barrier function and not influenced by other factors such as tear volume, osmolarity, or viscosity [103].
- It is fast and easy: the test can be performed in a few minutes with minimal training required for the operator [103].
- It is safe: the dye used in the test is typically administered in low doses and has a low risk of adverse reactions [103].
- It is reliable: the test has high repeatability, meaning that results can be reproduced consistently over time and across different operators [101, 103].
- It is dynamic: it can be used to monitor changes in corneal permeability over time, providing valuable information about disease progression or response to treatment [103].
- It is predictive: the test can indicate risk factors or prognosis for DED, allowing for early intervention and better management of the disease [103].
- It is responsive: changes in corneal permeability measured by fluorophotometry can reflect the effects of treatment, allowing for more precise and personalized treatment plans [108].

However, it also has some limitations:

- It requires specialized equipment: It is an expensive device that may not be widely available in clinical settings.
- It requires careful calibration: Before each measurement, the device needs to be adjusted according to ambient light conditions, background fluorescence, and patient characteristics such as pupil size, iris color, and refractive error [109].
- It requires standardized protocol: There are many variables that can affect this method such as dye concentration, volume, and instillation method; time interval between instillation and measurement; and number and duration of measurements. These variables need to be controlled and reported for accurate interpretation and comparison of data [110].
- It may cause discomfort: some patients may experience a burning sensation, tearing, or blurred vision after fluorescein instillation; these effects usually subside within minutes but may interfere with patient compliance or cooperation.

7.3 Potential role in future research and clinical practice

It can be used to evaluate the safety of contact lens wear. By measuring the corneal epithelial permeability and tear film thickness, it can detect changes in the ocular surface associated with contact lens wear, which can inform the development of safer and more effective contact lenses [111]. It can also be used to evaluate the efficacy of new drug candidates for DED by measuring the drug penetration through the cornea and the ocular surface, and it can provide insights into the drug's pharmacokinetics and bioavailability, which are crucial factors in determining the efficacy of topical ocular treatments.

Below are a few examples of how clinicians utilize fluorophotometry in the management of DED:

- Management of DED patients: It may be useful clinically because an increased corneal uptake of fluorescein reveals subtle damage to the corneal epithelium [98]. Its measurements of the penetration of fluorescein across the corneal epithelium could be of value in diagnosing or monitoring DED [103]. It has been investigated whether fluorophotometry correlated with previously established DED diagnostic tests and whether it could serve as a novel objective metric to evaluate DED [108].

- Evaluation of treatment effectiveness: It can be used to monitor the effectiveness of treatments aimed at improving tear film stability and corneal integrity, such as artificial tears, punctal occlusion, and topical medications. Measuring the rate of tear turnover and corneal permeability before and after treatment, it can help determine if the treatment is working as intended [103].

- Assessment of contact lens safety: It can be used to assess the safety of contact lens wear by measuring the corneal epithelial permeability and tear film thickness. These measurements can help identify changes in the ocular surface associated with contact lens wear, which can inform decisions about contact lens selection and management [111].

- Research: It is also used in research settings to investigate the underlying causes of DED and to evaluate new treatments. The quantitative measurements provided by fluorophotometry are useful for assessing treatment efficacy and for monitoring changes in tear film stability and corneal integrity over time [103].

In conclusion, fluorophotometry is a promising noninvasive technique that can provide objective and quantitative information about various aspects of DED, including corneal epithelial integrity and permeability, tear film stability, tear turnover rate, aqueous humor flow rate, and blood-retinal barrier integrity. It can be used to monitor changes in corneal permeability over time, evaluate risk factors or prognosis for DED, develop personalized treatment plans, investigate the pathophysiology of DED, and develop new treatments. However, careful calibration and specialized equipment are required before use.

8. Fluorescein corneography

Fluorescein corneography (FCG) (**Figure 6**) is a cutting-edge technique that has been developed to detect punctate epithelial erosions (PEE) with great precision.

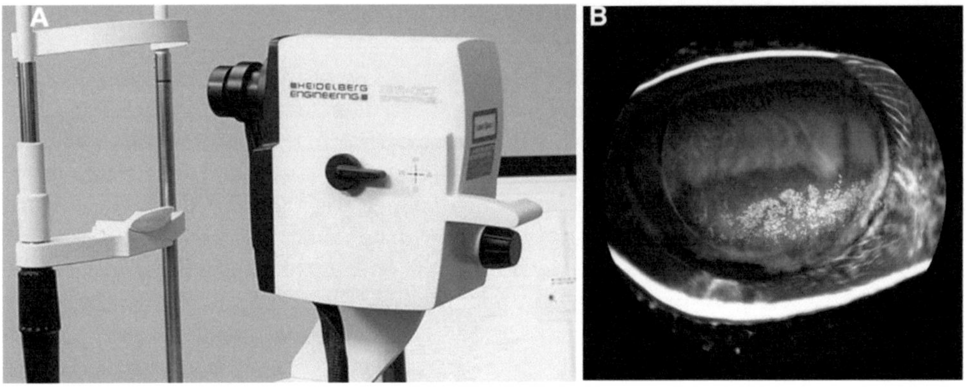

Figure 6.
(A) Fluorescein CorneoGraphy captures corneal epithelium fluorescein staining patterns. (B) Distribution of fluorescein stain in the tear film.

The technique utilizes a repurposed imaging system, the Heidelberg Spectralis II OCT with fluorescein angiography function, to capture the corneal epithelium staining patterns. The OCT-fluorescein angiography (FA) system is highly effective in providing robust detection of PEE in patients with DED [112].

8.1 Principles and applications

The principle behind FCG is to utilize the advanced capabilities of the Spectralis optical coherence tomography (OCT) system with fluorescein angiography (FA) function to visualize corneal epithelium staining patterns. The Spectralis imaging system has advantages over typical imaging with a cobalt-blue filter, as it uses a 490 nm excitation laser that enables superior excitation of fluorescein and more detailed imaging of the corneal surface. Additionally, the device uses an appropriate barrier filter to enable specific imaging of fluorescein emission around 525 nm [112].

To perform FCG, the inferior lid of the imaged eye is gently pulled down, and 2 microliters of 0.25% fluorescein sodium are instilled on the patient's lower tarsal conjunctiva using a micropipette. One minute after fluorescein instillation, an ocular wash using sterile PBS is performed using the same micropipette. This is done by asking the patient to incline their head to the contralateral side of the eye of interest, and 300 μL of sterile PBS is instilled through a micropipette, aiming at the ocular surface from the lateral sides in order to reduce fluorescein pooling and debris/tear film on the surface [112].

To obtain a complete corneal area visualization, the image frame is focused on a midpoint between the lacrimal caruncle and the corneal limbus while maintaining a thorough view of the corneal epithelium from limbus to limbus. The lens is focused on the corneal epithelium in such a way that both the central and peripheral epithelium are clearly visualized in their totality. The sensitivity knob is kept constant during imaging, with minute compensation for maximal clarity [112].

Some applications of FCG include:

- Diagnosis of PEE: It is a highly sensitive and accurate method for detecting PEE, which is a common sign of DED. This technique can provide clinicians with a standardized methodology for robust detection of PEE.

- Evaluation of the effectiveness of DED treatments: It can be used to evaluate the effectiveness of different DED treatments by monitoring changes in corneal staining patterns over time.

- Research studies: It can be utilized in research studies to investigate the pathophysiology of DED and to evaluate the efficacy of potential new treatments.

- Evaluation of corneal epithelial damage: It can be used to evaluate the extent of corneal epithelial damage in patients with other corneal disorders, such as corneal abrasions or infections.

- Screening tool for DED: It can be used as a screening tool for DED, especially in patients with light-colored irises who may not show typical signs of the condition.

8.2 Advantages and limitations

- Ability to focus on all regions of the cornea in one image.

- High contrast visualization.

- High sensitivity in detecting corneal staining.

- Particularly effective for light-colored iris patients.

- Standardized methodology for robust detection of PEE.

- Sensitive, rigorous and reproducible.

- Suitable for clinical and research practices.

- Commercially available.

- Safe and painless.

Nonetheless, it comes with certain constraints:

- Patient compliance for a perfectly centered image: The FCG standard operative procedure requires the patient to be compliant in achieving a perfectly centered image, which can be challenging for some patients.

- Need for external fixating light and second assistant: The OCT device used in the procedure requires an external fixating light to aid patients in centration, and a second assistant is needed to obtain a lid aperture, which may increase the complexity and length of the procedure.

- It may not be covered by insurance for DED diagnosis.

8.3 Potential role in future research and clinical practice

FCG has emerged as a crucial diagnostic tool that plays a pivotal role in unraveling the intricate pathophysiology of DED through its ability to generate high-resolution, real-time images of the corneal epithelium staining patterns, and it enables researchers to gain valuable insights into its underlying mechanisms. As a result, it holds significant potential for facilitating future research efforts aimed at enhancing our understanding of the etiology and management of DED [112].

Furthermore, it provides a means to obtain intricate images of the corneal epithelium staining patterns, which can be utilized to identify the underlying causes of the condition and unlock new potential treatment options. In addition, it can provide an objective way of assessing the effectiveness of different treatment modalities for DED, including topical eye drops, artificial tears, and other therapies. By monitoring changes in corneal staining patterns over time, FCG can serve as a sensitive and reliable metric to track disease progression and evaluate the response to different treatments. This information can provide clinicians and researchers with valuable insights into the efficacy of different interventions [112].

In clinical practice, it can be used to diagnose and monitor PEE, providing clinicians with a standardized and highly sensitive methodology for detecting PEE. Additionally, it can be used as a screening tool for DED, especially in patients with light-colored irises who may not show typical signs of the condition. Furthermore, FCG can be used to evaluate the effectiveness of different DED treatments by monitoring changes in corneal staining patterns over time [112].

In summary, FCG is an effective technique that has high sensitivity and accuracy in detecting PEE, which is a frequent sign of DED. FCG has considerable potential to aid future research endeavors focused on improving our comprehension of the causes and treatment of DED. Providing detailed images of the corneal epithelium staining patterns, it can help identify the root causes of the condition and pave the way for novel therapeutic interventions.

9. Conclusion

The various corneal imaging techniques available provide valuable diagnostic and management tools for ocular surface conditions, particularly DED. Each technique has its strengths and limitations, and a combination of tools can provide a more complete evaluation of the ocular surface. As technology continues to improve, these imaging techniques hold great potential for advancing our understanding of ocular surface diseases and developing new treatments. In clinical practice, utilizing a variety of imaging techniques can improve the accuracy of diagnosis and individualize treatment plans for patients with ocular surface conditions. Overall, these imaging techniques offer a promising future for improving the care of patients with DED and other ocular surface conditions.

Author details

Robby Mattes, Marcela Huertas-Bello and Alfonso L. Sabater*
Bascom Palmer Eye Institute, Miami, USA

*Address all correspondence to: asabater@med.miami.edu

References

[1] Kaur K, Gurnani B. Slit-lamp biomicroscope. In: StatPearls. Treasure Island (FL): StatPearls Publishing; 4 May 2023

[2] Szczesna-Iskander DH, Muzyka-Wozniak M, Llorens QC. The efficacy of ocular surface assessment approaches in evaluating dry eye treatment with artificial tears. Scientific Reports. 2022;**12**:21835. DOI: 10.1038/s41598-022-26327-3

[3] Shu X, Wang J, Hu L. A review of functional slit lamp biomicroscopy. Eye and vision (London, England). 2019;**6**:15. DOI: 10.1186/s40662-019-0140-7

[4] Sall K, Foulks GN, Pucker AD, Ice KL, Zink RC, Magrath G. Validation of a modified National eye Institute grading scale for corneal fluorescein staining. Clinical Ophthalmology. 2023;**17**:757-767. DOI: 10.2147/OPTH.S398843

[5] Begley CG, Caffery B, Chalmers RL, et al. Review and analysis of grading scales for ocular surface staining. The Ocular Surface. 2019;**17**(2):208-220. DOI: 10.1016/j.jtos.2019.01.004

[6] Singh RB, Liu L, Anchouche S, et al. Ocular redness - I: Etiology, pathogenesis, and assessment of conjunctival hyperemia. The Ocular Surface. 2021;**21**:134-144. DOI: 10.1016/j.jtos.2021.05.003

[7] Milner MS, Beckman KA, Luchs JI, et al. Dysfunctional tear syndrome: Dry eye disease and associated tear film disorders - new strategies for diagnosis and treatment. Current Opinion in Ophthalmology. 2017;**27 Suppl 1**(Suppl 1):3-47. DOI: 10.1097/01.icu.0000512373.81749.b7

[8] Baghdasaryan E, Feldman BH, Bunya VY, Woodward MA, Ahmad S. Dry eye syndrome. American Academy of Ophthalmology. 2023;**12**(1):1-10

[9] De Silva MEH, Zhang AC, Karahalios A, Chinnery HR, Downie LE. Laser scanning in vivo confocal microscopy (IVCM) for evaluating human corneal sub-basal nerve plexus parameters: Protocol for a systematic review. BMJ Open. 2017;**7**(11):e018646. DOI: 10.1136/bmjopen-2017-018646

[10] Patel DV, Zhang J, McGhee CNJ. In vivo confocal microscopy of the inflamed anterior segment: A review of clinical and research applications. Clinical & Experimental Ophthalmology. 2019;**47**(3):334-345

[11] Simsek C, Karalezli A, Dogru M, et al. In vivo confocal microscopy evaluation in dry eye and related diseases. Current Ophthalmology Reports. 2019;7(3):187-195. DOI: 10.1007/s40135-019-00216-x

[12] Akhlaq A, Colón C, Cavalcanti BM, et al. Density and distribution of dendritiform cells in the peripheral cornea of healthy subjects using in vivo confocal microscopy. Cornea. 2022;**41**(10):1310-1317. DOI: 10.1097/ICO.0000000000002878

[13] Zhao H, Chen JY, Wang YQ, Lin ZR, Wang S. In vivo confocal microscopy evaluation of meibomian gland dysfunction in dry eye patients with different symptoms. Chinese Medical Journal. 2016;**129**(21):2617-2622. DOI: 10.4103/0366-6999.192782

[14] Kheirkhah A, Rahimi Darabad R, Cruzat A, et al. Corneal epithelial immune dendritic cell alterations in subtypes of

DED: A pilot in vivo confocal microscopic study. Investigative Ophthalmology & Visual Science. 2015;**56**(12):7179. DOI: 10.1167/iovs.15-17433

[15] Barros A, Lozano-Sanroma J, Queiruga-Piñeiro J, et al. Recovery of corneal innervation after treatment in dry eye disease: A confocal microscopy study. Journal of Clinical Medicine. 2023;**12**(5):1841. DOI: 10.3390/jcm12051841

[16] Pflugfelder SC, Nettune GR. Ocular Surface Disease: Cornea, Conjunctiva and Tear Film. London: Elsevier; 2013

[17] Daull P, Feraille L, Elena PP, Garrigue JS. Comparison of the anti-inflammatory effects of artificial tears in a rat model of corneal scraping. Journal of Ocular Pharmacology and Therapeutics. 2016;**32**(2):99-107

[18] Iaccheri B, Torroni G, Cerquaglia A, et al. Evaluation of warm compresses and topical cyclosporine treatment in meibomian gland dysfunction by confocal scanning laser microscopy. European Journal of Ophthalmology. 2023;**33**(2):881-889. DOI: 10.1177/11206721221128995

[19] Cruzat A, Qazi Y, Hamrah P. In vivo confocal microscopy of corneal nerves in health and disease. The Ocular Surface. 2017;**15**(1):15-47. DOI: 10.1016/j.jtos.2016.09.004

[20] Qazi Y, Kheirkhah A, Blackie C, et al. In vivo detection of clinically non-apparent ocular surface inflammation in patients with meibomian gland dysfunction-associated refractory dry eye symptoms: A pilot study. Eye. 2015;**29**(8):1099-1110

[21] Daull P, Feraille L, Elena PP, Garrigue JS. Comparison of the anti-inflammatory effects of artificial tears in a rat model of corneal scraping. Journal of Ocular Pharmacology and Therapeutics. 2016;**32**(2):108-117. DOI: 10.1089/jop.2015.0054

[22] Villani E, Mantelli F, Nucci P. In-vivo confocal microscopy of the ocular surface: Ocular allergy and dry eye. Current Opinion in Allergy and Clinical Immunology. 2013;**13**(5):569-576. DOI: 10.1097/ACI.0b013e328364ec92

[23] Zhang Y, Li J, Zhang X, et al. In vivo confocal microscopic evaluation of corneal dendritic cell density and subbasal nerve plexus changes in patients with thyroid-associated Ophthalmopathy. Frontiers in Medicine (Lausanne). 2021;**8**:578233. DOI: 10.3389/fmed.2021.578233

[24] Hwang J, Dermer H, Galor A. Can in vivo confocal microscopy differentiate between sub-types of dry eye disease? A review. Clinical & Experimental Ophthalmology. 2021;**49**(4):373-387. DOI: 10.1111/ceo.1392

[25] Nanji AA, Mercado C, Galor A, Dubovy S, Karp CL. Updates in ocular surface tumor diagnostics. International Ophthalmology Clinics. 2017;**57**(3):47-62. DOI: 10.1097/IIO.0000000000000174

[26] Aggarwal S, Kheirkhah A, Cavalcanti BM, Cruzat A, Jamali A, Hamrah P. Correlation of corneal immune cell changes with clinical severity in DED: An in vivo confocal microscopy study. Cornea. 2020;**39**(5):565-571

[27] Weiner G. Dry eye disease. American Academy of Ophthalmology. EyeNet Magazine. 2018;**22**(4):37-43

[28] Bartlett J, Keith M, Sudharshan L, Snedecor S. Associations between signs and symptoms of DED: A systematic

review of correlations among subjective and objective clinical tests. Clinical Ophthalmology. 2015;**9**:1719-1730. DOI: 10.2147/OPTH.S89700

[29] Liang QF, Gao C, Liang H, Du XH, Wang NL, Labbe A. In vivo confocal microscopy evaluation of meibomian glands in meibomian gland dysfunction patients. Chinese Journal of Ophthalmology. 2016;**52**(9):649-656. DOI: 10.3760/cma.j.issn.0412-4081.2016.09.004

[30] Ling J, Chan BCL, Tsang MSM, et al. Current advances in mechanisms and treatment of DED: Toward anti-inflammatory and immunomodulatory therapy and traditional Chinese medicine. Frontiers in Medicine. 2022;**8**(815075):1-19

[31] Ramírez BE, Sánchez A, Herreras JM, et al. Stem cell therapy for corneal epithelium regeneration following good manufacturing and clinical procedures. BioMed Research International. 2015;**2015**(408495):1-12. DOI: 10.1155/2015/408495

[32] Villani E, Baudouin C, Efron N, et al. In vivo confocal microscopy of the ocular surface: From bench to bedside. Current Eye Research. 2014;**39**(3):213-231. DOI: 10.3109/02713683.2013.842592

[33] Fercher AF, Drexler W, Hitzenberger CK, Lasser T. Optical coherence tomography - principles and applications. Reports on Progress in Physics. 2003;**66**(2):239-303. DOI: 10.1088/0034-4885/66/2/204

[34] Fercher AF. Optical coherence tomography – Development, principles, applications [in German]. Zeitschrift für Medizinische Physik. 2010;**20**(1):6-16

[35] Shan J, DeBoer C, Xu BY. Anterior segment optical coherence tomography: Applications for clinical care and scientific research. Asia-Pacific Journal of Ophthalmology (Philadelphia). 2019;**8**(2):146-157. DOI: 10.22608/APO.201910

[36] Xu W, Wang H. Using beam-offset optical coherence tomography to reconstruct backscattered photon profiles in scattering media. Biomedical Optics Express (Optica Publishing Group). 2022;**13**(11):6124-6135. Published 2022 Oct 31. DOI: 10.1364/BOE.469082

[37] Pircher M, Zawadzki RJ. Review of adaptive optics OCT (AO-OCT): Principles and applications for retinal imaging [invited]. Biomedical Optics Express. 2017;**8**(5):2536-2562. DOI: 10.1364/BOE.8.002536

[38] Aumann S, Donner S, Fischer J, Müller F. Optical coherence tomography (OCT): Principle and technical realization. In: Drexler W, Fujimoto JG, editors. Optical Coherence Tomography: Technology and Applications. 3rd ed. Cham: Springer; 2019. pp. 59-98. DOI: 10.1007/978-3-030-16638-0_3

[39] Fujimoto JG, Schmitt J, Swanson E, Aguirre AD, Jang IK. The development of optical coherence tomography. In: Drexler W, Fujimoto JG, editors. Optical Coherence Tomography: Technology and Applications. 3rd ed. Cham: Springer; 2019. pp. 1-57. DOI: 10.1007/978-3-030-25711-8_1

[40] Themes UFO. Introduction to Swept Source OCT. Ento Key. Published October 16 2017

[41] Wang X, Yuan X, Shi L. Optical coherence tomography—in situ and high-speed 3D imaging for laser materials processing. Light: Science & Applications. 2022;**11**(1):280. DOI: 10.1038/s41377-022-00981-8

[42] Park KS, Park E, Lee H, et al. Phase stable swept-source optical coherence tomography with active mode-locking

laser for contrast enhancements of retinal angiography. Scientific Reports. 2021;**11**(1):16636. DOI: 10.1038/s41598-021-95982-9

[43] Fujimoto JG. Optical coherence tomography (OCT) in ophthalmology: Introduction. Optics Express. 2009;**17**(5):3978-3979

[44] Levy A, Georgeon C, Knoeri J, et al. Corneal epithelial thickness mapping in the diagnosis of ocular surface disorders involving the corneal epithelium: A comparative study. Cornea. 2022;**41**(11):1353-1361. DOI: 10.1097/ICO.0000000000003012

[45] Costello F, Burton J. Retinal imaging with optical coherence tomography: A biomarker in multiple sclerosis? Eye and Brain. 2018;**10**:47-63

[46] Gallwas J, Turk L, Friese K, Dannecker C. Optical coherence tomography as a non-invasive imaging technique for preinvasive and invasive neoplasia of the uterine cervix. Ultrasound in Obstetrics & Gynecology. 2010;**36**(2):246-250. DOI: 10.1002/uog.7656

[47] Engineering H. Imaging that enlightens: Deeper insights into retinal structures with high-resolution OCT. The Ophthalmologist. 2022;**4**(2):12-15

[48] Boppart SA. Optical coherence tomography: Technology and applications for neuroimaging. Psychophysiology. 2003;**40**(4):529-541. DOI: 10.1111/1469-8986.00055

[49] Pennington LM, Smith B. OCT: What's under the Hood? This essential guide will help you understand the technology and how it supports clinical practice. Review of Optometry. 2021;**158**(9):40-47

[50] Shen Lee B, Kabat AG, Bacharach J, Karpecki P, Luchs J. Managing dry eye disease and facilitating realistic patient expectations: A review and appraisal of current therapies. Clinical Ophthalmology. 2020;**14**:119-126. DOI: 10.2147/OPTH.S228838

[51] Mazzarella J, Cole J. The anatomy of an OCT scan. Review of Optometry. 2015;**152**(9):36-42

[52] Spirn MJ, Feldman BH, Kozak A, Shah VA, Kim LA, Tripathy K, et al. Optical coherence tomography. American Academy of Ophthalmology. 2015;**122**(2):417-422

[53] Sissons B. What to know about OCT for macular degeneration. Medical News Today. May 19, 2022

[54] Tanasescu C, Wu KY, Bunya VY. Imaging modalities for dry eye disease. American Academy of Ophthalmology. October. 2019;**7**

[55] Edorh NA, El Maftouhi A, Djerada Z, Arndt C, Denoyer A. New model to better diagnose dry eye disease integrating OCT corneal epithelial mapping. The British Journal of Ophthalmology. 2022;**106**(11):1488-1495. DOI: 10.1136/bjophthalmol-2021-318826

[56] Sevgi DD, Ehlers JP. Advances in intraoperative OCT. Review of Ophthalmology. 2019;**26**(10):32-35

[57] Iftimia N, Hammer DX, Mujat M, Desphande V, Cizginer S, Brugge W. Optical coherence tomography imaging for cancer diagnosis and therapy guidance. En: Zhang YT et al., eds. 2009 Annual International Conference of the IEEE Engineering in Medicine and Biology Society; September 3-6; Minneapolis, MN. Piscataway: IEEE; 2009: 1460-1463

[58] Huang D, Swanson EA, Lin CP, et al. Optical coherence tomography. Science. 1991;**254**(5035):1178-1181. DOI: 10.1126/science.1957169

[59] Bouma BE, de Boer JF, Huang D, et al. Optical coherence tomography. Nature Reviews Methods Primers. 2022;**2**:79. DOI: 10.1038/s43586-022-00162-2

[60] Gordon AY, Jayagopal A. Engineering of nanoscale contrast agents for optical coherence tomography. Journal of Nanomedicine & Nanotechnology. 2014;**Suppl 5**:004. DOI: 10.4172/2157-7439.S5-004

[61] Bai Y, Ngo W, Nichols JJ. Characterization of the thickness of the tear film lipid layer using high resolution microscopy. The Ocular Surface. 2019;**17**(2):356-359

[62] Isreb MA, Greiner JV, Korb DR, et al. Correlation of lipid layer thickness measurements with fluorescein tear film break-up time and Schirmer's test. Eye. 2003;**17**(1):79-83

[63] Sweeney DF, Millar TJ, Raju SR. Tear film stability: A review. Experimental Eye Research. 2013;**117**:28-38

[64] Zhang J, Wu Z, Sun L, Liu XH. Function and morphology of the meibomian glands using a LipiView interferometer in rotating shift medical staff. Journal of Ophthalmology (Hindawi). 2020;**2020**:3275143. Published 2020 Aug 17. DOI: 10.1155/2020/3275143

[65] Lee JM, Jeon YJ, Kim KY, Hwang KY, Kwon YA, Koh K. Ocular surface analysis: A comparison between the LipiView® II and IDRA®. European Journal of Ophthalmology (EuropePMC). Sep 2021;**31**(5):2300-2306. DOI: 10.1177/1120672120969035

[66] Lee Y, Hyon JY, Jeon HS. Characteristics of dry eye patients with thick tear film lipid layers evaluated by a LipiView II interferometer. Graefe's Archive for Clinical and Experimental Ophthalmology=Albrecht Von Graefes ArchivFur Klinische Und Experimentelle Ophthalmologie. 2021;**259**(5):1235-1241

[67] Mainstone JC, Bruce AS, Golding TR. Tear meniscus measurement in the diagnosis of dry eye. Current Eye Research. 1996;**15**(6):653-661. DOI: 10.3109/02713689609017639

[68] Ji YW, Lee J, Lee H, Seo KY, Kim EK, Kim TI. Automated measurement of tear film dynamics and lipid layer thickness for assessment of Non-Sjögren dry eye syndrome with meibomian gland dysfunction. Cornea (Wolters Kluwer). 2017;**36**(2):176-182. DOI: 10.1097/ICO.0000000000001101

[69] Lemp MA. Tear Film: Basic and Clinical Aspects. Marcel Dekker; 1995

[70] Mishima S, Maurice DM. The oily layer of the tear film and evaporation from the corneal surface. Experimental Eye Research. 1961;**1**(3):39-45. DOI: 10.1016/s0014-4835(61)80009-3

[71] Guillon M, Maissa C, Wong S. Eyelid-induced perturbations of the tear film: A review. Contact Lens & Anterior Eye. 2012;**35**(2):77-82. DOI: 10.1016/j.clae.2011.10.006

[72] Finis D, Ackermann P, Pischel N, et al. Evaluation of lipid layer thickness measurement of the tear film as a diagnostic tool for Meibomian gland dysfunction. Cornea. 2013;**32**(12):1549-1553. DOI: 10.1097/ICO.0b013e31829c4163

[73] Bron AJ, Tiffany JM. The contribution of meibomian disease to dry eye. Ocular Surface. 2011;**9**(3):149-158

[74] Yokoi N, Bron AJ, Tiffany JM. Reflectivity of the surface lipid layer on the exposed meibomian gland orifice. Ocular Surface. 2017;**15**(4):683-688

[75] King-Smith PE, Hinel EA, Nichols JJ. Application of a novel interferometric method to investigate the relation between lipid layer thickness and tear film thinning. Investigative Ophthalmology & Visual Science. 2010;**51**(5):2418-2423. DOI: 10.1167/iovs.09-4387

[76] Goto E et al. Tear evaporation rates in Sjögren syndrome and non-Sjögren dry eye patients. American Journal of Ophthalmology. 2007;**144**(5):744-748

[77] Tomlinson A et al. Tear film osmolarity: Determination of a referent for dry eye diagnosis. Investigative Ophthalmology & Visual Science. 2006;**47**(10):4309-4315

[78] Arita R et al. Meibomian gland dysfunction and contact lens discomfort. Eye & Contact Lens. 2017;**43**(6):352-356

[79] Choi W et al. Evaluation of lipid layer thickness measurement of the tear film as a diagnostic tool for meibomian gland dysfunction. Cornea. 2017;**36**(5):517-522

[80] Wolffsohn JS et al. Effect of time of day and instruction on repeatability of lipid layer thickness measurements. Contact Lens & Anterior Eye. 2012;**35**(6):281-285

[81] Sullivan BD et al. Androgen deficiency, Meibomian gland dysfunction, and evaporative dry eye. Annals of the New York Academy of Sciences. 2002;**966**:211-222

[82] Kanclerz P, Khoramnia R, Wang X. Current developments in corneal topography and tomography. Diagnostics (Basel, Switzerland). 2021;**11**(8):1466. Published 2021 Aug 13. DOI: 10.3390/diagnostics11081466

[83] Yilmaz S, Yuksel T, Maden A. Corneal topographic changes after four types of pterygium surgery. Journal of Refractive Surgery. 2008;**24**(2):160-165. DOI: 10.3928/1081597X-20080201-06

[84] Sridhar U, Tripathy K. Corneal topography. In: StatPearls [Internet]. StatPearls: Treasure Island (FL); 2023

[85] Feldman BH, Prakash G, Bunya VY, Akkara JD, Bernfeld E, Chen M. Corneal topography. In: American Academy of Ophthalmology. Assigned status Up to Date by Masako Chen, MD on March 12. 2023

[86] Oliveira CM, Ribeiro C, Franco S. Corneal imaging with slit-scanning and Scheimpflug imaging techniques. Clinical and Experimental Optometry (Wiley Online Library). 2011;**94**(1):33-42. DOI: 10.1111/j.1444-0938.2010.00509.x

[87] Martin R. Cornea and anterior eye assessment with placido-disc keratoscopy, slit scanning evaluation topography and scheimpflug imaging tomography. Indian Journal of Ophthalmology (Wolters Kluwer). 2018;**66**(3):360-366. DOI: 10.4103/ijo.IJO_850_17

[88] Fan R, Chan TC, Prakash G, Jhanji V. Applications of corneal topography and tomography: A review. Clinical & Experimental Ophthalmology (Wiley Online Library). 2018;**46**(2):133-146. DOI: 10.1111/ceo.13136

[89] Liu Z, Huang AJ, Pflugfelder SC. Evaluation of corneal thickness and topography in normal eyes using the Orbscan corneal topography system. British Journal of Ophthalmology. 1999;**83**(7):774-778. DOI: 10.1136/bjo.83.7.774

[90] Guven S. The repeatability of corneal topography measurements in severe dry eye disease. BMC Ophthalmology. 2022;**22**(1):306. Published 2022 Jul 15. DOI: 10.1186/s12886-022-02534-4

[91] Doğan AŞ, Gürdal C, Köylü MT. Does dry eye affect repeatability of corneal topography measurements? Türk Oftalmoloji Dergisi. 2018:57-60 Published online April 27

[92] Chen A, Lin B, Lin S. How to interpret corneal topography: 5 clinical uses. EyeGuru. Published in 2019

[93] Mohammadi SF, Khorrami-Nejad M, Hamidirad M. Posterior corneal astigmatism: A review article. Optometry and Vision Science. 2019;**96**(9):677-684. DOI: 10.1097/OPX.0000000000001421

[94] Lee JS, Jun I, Kim EK, Seo KY, Kim TI. Clinical accuracy of an advanced corneal topographer with tear-film analysis in functional and structural evaluation of dry eye disease. Seminars in Ophthalmology (Taylor & Francis). 2020;**35**(2):134-140. DOI: 10.1080/08820538.2020.1755321

[95] Buehren T, Collins MJ, Iskander DR, Davis B, Lingelbach B. The stability of corneal topography in the post-blink interval. Cornea (Wolters Kluwer). 2001;**20**(8):826-833. DOI: 10.1097/00003226-200111000-00010

[96] Yang HK, Che SA, Hyon JY, Han SB. Integration of artificial intelligence into the approach for diagnosis and monitoring of DED. Diagnostics. 2022;**12**(12):3167

[97] Gu H, Guo Y, Gu L, Wei A. Deep learning for identifying corneal diseases from ocular surface slit-lamp photographs. Scientific Reports. 2020;**10**(1):1-9

[98] Roberts CJ, Mahmoud AM, Bons JP, et al. Introduction of two novel stiffness parameters and interpretation of air puff-induced biomechanical deformation parameters with a dynamic Scheimpflug Analyzer. Journal of Refractive Surgery. 2017;**33**(4):266-273

[99] Doctor K, Vunnava KP, Shroff R, et al. Simplifying and understanding various topographic indices for keratoconus using Scheimpflug based topographers. Indian Journal of Ophthalmology. 2020;**68**(12):2732-2743. DOI: 10.4103/ijo.IJO_2111_20

[100] Ozcura F, Aydin S, Helvaci MR. Ocular surface disease index for the diagnosis of dry eye syndrome. Ocular Immunology and Inflammation (Taylor & Francis). 2007;**15**(5):389-393. DOI: 10.1080/09273940701486803

[101] Mochizuki H, Yamada M, Hatou S, Tsubota K. Turnover rate of tear-film lipid layer determined by fluorophotometry. British Journal of Ophthalmology. 2009;**93**(11):1535-1538. DOI: 10.1136/bjo.2008.156828

[102] Nagaya T, Nakamura YA, Choyke PL, Kobayashi H. Current and new fluorescent probes for fluorescence-guided surgery. In: Hoffman RM, Bouvet M, editors. Strategies for Curative Fluorescence-Guided Surgery of Cancer. ScienceDirect. Academic Press; 2020. pp. 75-114. DOI: 10.1016/B978-0-12-812576-2.00006-9

[103] Fahim MM, Haji S, Koonapareddy CV, Fan VC, Asbell PA. Fluorophotometry as a diagnostic tool for the evaluation of DED. BMC Ophthalmology. 2006;**6**:20. Published 2006 Jul 18. DOI: 10.1186/1471-2415-6-20

[104] Wang Y, Cao G, Wen L, et al. A new optical model for photomultiplier tubes. European Physical Journal C.

2022;**82**(329). DOI: 10.1140/epjc/s10052-022-10288-y

[105] Goldschmidt MC. Biosensors – Scope in microbiological analysis. In: Batt CA, Tortorello ML, editors. Encyclopedia of Food Microbiology. 2nd ed. ScienceDirect. Elsevier, Academic Press; 2014. pp. 274-287. DOI: 10.1016/B978-0-12-384730-0.00041-0

[106] Srinivas SP, Goyal A, Talele DP, et al. Corneal epithelial permeability to fluorescein in humans by a multi-drop method. PLoS One. 2018;**13**(6):e0198831

[107] Sorbara L, Simpson T, Vaccari S, Jones L, Fonn D. Tear turnover rate is reduced in patients with symptomatic dry eye. Contact Lens and Anterior Eye. 2004;**27**(1):15-20

[108] Fujitani K, Gadaria N, Lee KI, Barry B, Asbell P. Corneal permeability changes in DED: An observational study. BMC Ophthalmology. 2016;**16**(1):68. DOI: 10.1186/s12886-016-0231-3

[109] Toris CB, Gagrani M, Ghate D. Current methods and new approaches to assess aqueous humor dynamics. Ophthalmology Glaucoma. 2021;**4**(1):1-10

[110] Conway BP. Technical variables in vitreous fluorophotometry. Graefe's Archive for Clinical and Experimental Ophthalmology. 1985;**222**(4-5):194-201. DOI: 10.1007/BF02133673

[111] McNamara NA, Polse KA, Bonanno JA. Fluorophotometry in contact lens research: The next step. Optometry and Vision Science. 1998;**75**(5):357-364. DOI: 10.1097/00006324- 199805000-00020

[112] Soifer M, Azar NS, Blanco R, Mousa HM, Ghalibafan S, Tovar A, et al. Fluorescein CorneoGraphy (FCG): Use of a repurposed fluorescein imaging technique to objectively standardize corneal staining. The Ocular Surface. 2023;**27**(1):77-79. DOI: 10.1016/j.jtos.2022.11.010

Section 4

Updates on Management

Chapter 6

Intense Regulated Pulsed Light (IRPL) for Dry Eye Treatment

Eduardo Rojas Alvarez and Naima Pino Urias

Abstract

IRPL was traditionally used for the treatment of a variety of dermatological diseases such as rosacea. However, third-generation equipment was created specifically for periocular application with multiple homogeneously sculpted pulses "It is the only IRPL device medically certified to treat Meibomian Gland Dysfunction." Several hypotheses or effects of how the device works have been proposed. Ablation of the small telangiectatic vessels around the eyelid, elimination or reduction of the ectoparasite Demodex, which resides in the meibomian glands and consumes meibum secretions in patients who have rosacea, photomodulation of the glands stimulates cellular activity, improving the micro and macro structure of the meibomian glands. In addition, the modification would decrease the inflammation surrounding them.

Keywords: regulated intense pulsed light, dry eye, meibomian glands, dry rosacea, dry eye treatment

1. Introduction

Dry eye syndrome (DES) due to meibomian gland dysfunction (MGD) is a chronic alteration manifested by both quantitative and qualitative changes of the meibum, affecting the tear film and causing ocular irritation, inflammation, and/or pain [1]. According to Rouen, the worldwide prevalence rate of the syndrome is between 5% and 50%, but it can even reach 75%, depending on the geographical region and the age of the person, being more frequent in adults over 40 years old, predominantly in women. 2.7% of those suffering from DES are adults between 18 and 45 years of age [2].

The basic treatment for people suffering from DES consists of the administration of artificial tears, the use of warm compresses, changes in the usual diet, increasing the intake of omega-3 oils, and the use of antibiotics and/or topical corticosteroids. However, despite the large number of options for management, in most cases, patients are not completely satisfied, causing discomfort and difficulties in their daily lives, which leads to the search for other therapies [3].

Intense regulated pulsed light (IRPL) is a digital device traditionally used for the treatment of a variety of dermatological conditions such as rosacea. However, third-generation equipment was created specifically for periocular application with multiple homogeneously sculpted pulses. IRPL uses a xenon flash lamp to emit wavelengths of light from 400 to 1200 nm. When placed over the light, a filter restricts the wavelength to the visible light range of 500 nm. When applied to the skin, this 500 nm light allows the blood vessels to capture the light and coagulation to occur, and eventually, they close [4].

IRPL is a relatively new therapy, which as of 2017, the Tear Film and Ocular Surface Society, included within the alternatives for the management of DES. However, the use of IRPL was well recognized in the field of dermatology for the treatment of dermal conditions such as rosacea, cavernous hemangiomas, and hypertrichosis, among others [5]. Its mechanism of action is developed through the uptake of light by the oxyhemoglobin present in red blood cells, generating heat and activating the coagulation process that induces thrombosis of blood vessels [6].

2. Development

IRPL was proposed as a therapy for DES when it was discovered by chance that patients who were being treated for rosacea and who also suffered from this syndrome, with intense pulsed light, improved their symptomatology during the application of this technology. In order to be able to use and disseminate the efficacy of the use of IPLR in DES, it is essential to describe the effects it causes, and the improvement perceived by the patients after the therapy. The epidemiological characteristics of DES, such as the factors that predispose to its development, are unknown in our environment. Variables such as age, sex, systemic diseases, including those of autoimmune origin (rheumatoid arthritis, Sjögren's syndrome), diabetes, rosacea; ocular pathology: glaucoma, conjunctivitis; and to establish vulnerable groups that suffer from DES.

2.1 Definition

IRPL was traditionally used for the treatment of a variety of dermatological diseases such as rosacea. However, third-generation equipment was created specifically for periocular application with multiple homogeneously sculpted pulses, "It is the only IRPL device medically certified to treat GMD. Within its fundamental parameters, it includes an area to be treated of 7.5 cm2 with a wavelength between 580 and 1200 nm, at temperatures ranging from -5°C to + 65°C" [3, 7].

2.2 Technical specifications

Features	IRPL
Dimensions: length x width x height	345 x 320 x 440 mm
Weight:	11.5 kg
Packaging dimensions: length x width x height	740 x 460 x 610 mm
Packaging weight:	17.5 kg
Noise level:	55 dBA
Energy consumption:	540 VA

DOI: http://dx.doi.org/10.5772/intechopen.110141

2.3 Mechanism of action

Several hypotheses or effects of how the device works have been proposed.

- Heat stimulation of the MG, with the aim of altering the physical properties of the meibum inside, causes it to become increasingly fluid. However, this theory is not very well accepted, as the effect of intense light on the temperature increase in the eyelid may be modest and transient [6].

- Ablation of the small telangiectatic vessels around the eyelid decreases local inflammation by reducing the levels of inflammatory mediators reaching the MG. It also provides a hypoxic environment, which has been found to be beneficial to the gland [6].

- Elimination or reduction of the ectoparasite Demodex, which resides in the meibomian glands and consumes meibum secretions in patients who have rosacea. In addition, the presence of the ectoparasite promotes a proinflammatory environment that affects the surface of the eyelid and then the eyeball. However, the Demodex exoskeleton could be vulnerable to the energy of the device, thus contributing to DES treatment [6].

- Photomodulation of the glands stimulates cellular activity, improving the micro and macro structure of the Meibomian glands. In addition, the modification would decrease the inflammation surrounding them [6].

- IRPL can stimulate the mitochondria in the tarsal plate, modifying their reagent production [6].

2.4 Method of application

- First, the entire region near the eyeball (lower and lateral skin) is cleaned, then both eyes are closed and a bilateral occluder is placed. Next, proceed to place gel all over the area where the treatment will be applied, starting from the temporal orbital region, inferior skin to the lower eyelids, and finally to the contralateral region [8].

- Then, five flashes should be applied, starting in the internal nasal region until reaching the temporal region, in both eyes, then the gel is removed from the face region and lidocaine in eye drops is instilled at the rate of one drop in both eyes. The examination is continued with the anterior biomicroscope and the MG expression is performed, previously applying topical anesthesia, located in the palpebral conjunctiva in the MG area, pressure is applied on the skin with the index finger close to the same gland to explore, for 30 seconds [8].

- The process should be repeated on both eyes and on the upper and lower eyelids. To do so, the patient should direct his gaze in a direction opposite to the eyelid being examined. Finally, the meibomian secretion located on the palpebral edges is cleaned [8].

2.5 Research carried out

IRPL as management for DES is a new treatment that is revolutionizing ophthalmic medicine, therefore, the studies consulted to perform the comparison of results include research developed in European countries, pioneers in this area of health.

In the first study conducted by Toyos in 2015, the treatment was performed on 78 patients (156 eyes) with dry eye syndrome (DES), caused by dysfunction of the meibomian glands (MGD), a statistically significant improvement in tear breakup time (TBUT) was observed from the beginning to the end of the treatment, 86% of the participants improved their TBUT in both eyes, in 9% no changes were evident and in 5% TBUT deteriorated in one of the eyes [4].

A second study conducted in 2020 by Vergés showed that 44 consecutive patients (88 eyes), ranging from 22 to 78 years, had significant improvements in single and total signs and symptoms. The most significant changes were seen in dryness, foreign body sensation, and pain. The OSDI questionnaire showed a significant decrease in total symptoms. The percentage of patients with a normal index improved from 23.8% (10 patients) at baseline to 80.9% (34 patients) at the last visit, after 23 weeks. Clinical signs also improved, by more than 90%, with telangiectasia and blepharitis standing out. No statistical differences were observed between age and sex. Clinical improvement started after the second and third weeks of IRPL application. Subsequently, the results remained stable until the last visit, after 11 weeks. No local, periocular, or systemic complications were reported [9].

In our study in Ecuador of 64 patients with diagnosis of DES, we performed three sessions of IRPL in the Exiláser Ophthalmologic Center. The majority of patients were male, a similar prevalence found in the study of evaluation of IRPL and the efficacy of meibomian gland expression in the relief of signs and symptoms by Dell, et al. with 58%, [10] unlike what was observed in the study conducted by Yun Tang et al. in 2020, in which the prevailing sex was female [11].

The average age of our study was 56 years, being the most frequent patients older than 58 years, and the ages of the universe were from 25 to 79 years [11]. In the first investigation in which the effects of IPRL for DES were studied by Toyos, McGill, and Briscoe, they obtained that the most frequent range was from 21 to 84 years, with a median of 54 [4]. In the work carried out by Yun Tang in order to study the main effects of IPRL, developed in China, the prevalent age range was from 23 to 86 years, with a median of 45 years [11]. In a review carried out in Mexico by Mendoza and Fortoul, they rightly mention that the prevalence of DES increases over the years, with 2.7% in people aged 18 to 34 years, to 18.6% in the population older than 75 years, justifying the higher percentage found in the present study [12].

Patient's profession is a variable that has also been related to the increased risk of DES, especially those who must remain for long periods of time in front of screens such as cell phones, telephones, and computers, among others, in addition, occupations that require exposure to toxic environmental factors such as carbon dioxide or carbon monoxide. In the course of the analysis of our research, it was found that most of the universe corresponds to other professions among which were drivers, health professionals, engineers, and architects, the same that are related to the established risk factors.

In the review carried out in Mexico, it was found that the permanent use of masks necessary to combat SARS-CoV-2 increases the risk of suffering DES, a preventive measure used in all the occupations mentioned [12]. In a study carried out in Cuba by Diburnet et al. 42% of the patients read excessively, corresponding in the study to teachers and students; it was also mentioned that 34% were exposed to digital media without blinking [7].

Regarding personal pathological antecedents, it was evidenced that more than half of the patients did not report the presence of any underlying systemic disease. However, arterial hypertension, type II diabetes mellitus, and autoimmune diseases such as systemic lupus erythematosus and Sjögren's syndrome were present. In addition, it was observed that a large percentage presented more than one particular pathology, among them thyroid disorders, especially hypothyroidism.

The risk factors established in several reviews for DES include systemic diseases, as indicated in the article by Rouen et al. published in 2018, in which autoimmune diseases, mainly Sjögren's syndrome, and chronic conditions, such as thyroid disorders, diabetes, rosacea, allergy, and conjunctivitis, are established as predisposing to the appearance of DES [2].

In a study conducted in Palestine during the period 2016 and 2017 by Shanti et al.; it was evidenced that 17% of the 769 participants reported having type II diabetes mellitus, while 20.9% reported having arterial hypertension [13]. It should be noted that the drugs used for these pathologies, such as antihypertensives, antihistamines, and diuretics, are factors associated with DES.

To finish with the personal history, in Ref. to the ophthalmologic, the reviewed bibliography mentions that surgeries or ocular lesions can influence the presence of DES [2]. The cases analyzed in our study did not have previous eye surgeries. However, ocular lesions were present, the most prevalent being a history of cataracts, followed by myopia and conjunctivitis.

DES significantly affects the daily lives of many people, especially in their daily activities. The main symptoms reported by patients who were seen at the Exiláser clinic during the period 2016–2021 were ocular pain, irritation on the ocular surface, and burning. The study conducted by Armas N. et al., in Cuba with a sample of 103 patients, determined that the main symptom presented by patients was ocular dryness at 64.1% followed by a gritty sensation at 59.2% and itching at 33% [14]. The study conducted by Perez MV. et al. at the University of Caracas in the year 2000 shows that the most frequent symptoms are ocular burning, foreign body sensation, and photophobia [15].

The results obtained show that the most prevalent sign was conjunctival hyperemia, followed by ocular dryness and irregularities of the palpebral edge, among which were trichiasis and telangiectasis, especially blepharitis. It should be mentioned that these signs decreased during the course of the IRPL sessions, the patients showed improvement in discomfort and it was demonstrated by the decrease in the irregularities of the palpebral rim.

The glandular expression before the IRPL sessions was predominantly granular/lumpy, followed by nontransparent fluid. After the IRPL sessions, nontransparent fluid predominated, followed by clear transparent fluid. However, granular glandular expression persisted in some patients.

In previous years, established treatments for this syndrome only included artificial tears and eye drops, which lubricated the ocular surface, reducing tear osmolarity and decreasing inflammation. The components of these substances are hyaluronic acid, carmellose, and polyacrylic acid. Eyelid hygiene also helps to control DES, using lotions and gels without preservatives, in addition to the use of warm compresses and massages, which help in cleansing and favor glandular expression [16]. However, despite all the therapies, people with DES did not show significant improvement.

In the article published in 2017 by Dell et al., which evaluates the efficacy of PLRI in relieving the signs and symptoms of DES due to meibomian gland dysfunction, they propose that the mechanism of action of this therapy is based on the transmitted energy ranging from 550 mm to 1200 mm, which is absorbed by the abnormal blood vessels and destroyed by thrombolysis [10]. The abnormal blood vessels, during the disease release inflammatory and proinflammatory substances, when they are destroyed, a large number of inflammation-causing substances decrease, which impairs the obstruction in the meibomian glands, being the main cause of DES.

Another hypothesis is the enhancement of the production of glandular expression, which decreases the bacterial load, especially mites (Demodex), after transferring heat to the eyelids and meibomian glands. In the study carried out by Miotto et al., they also mention that heat production destroys pigmented skin lesions, which has been the mechanism of action used in dermatological diseases such as rosacea, stating that the proposed mechanisms of action significantly increase the lipid levels of the lacrimal expression, which could increase the flow of secretion of the meibomian glands, and these effects would be cumulative, so that in the course of the three sessions, ocular improvement would be presented with greater duration, unlike empirical treatments [17].

The above is reflected in the level of pressure that had to be exerted for glandular expression before and after treatment. There was a predominance of severe pressure, before completing the IRPL sessions, and moderate pressure, followed by mild pressure after completing the treatment.

One of the most commonly used tools in the DES is the OSDI test, which evaluates 12 items, and after the answers, the degree of affectation in the person's daily life can be established. In this research, most of the participants presented a DES of moderate severity, followed by mild and finally a severe degree; the minority obtained a score lower than 12, similar results found in previously developed studies, for instance, the application of the OSDI test in Monterrey by Garza et al., in which they studied the prevalence, symptoms, and risk factors for diseases of the ocular surface, in the same, most of the participants, presented a score higher than 12.

The research conducted in 2015, by Gonzalez et al., aimed at validating the OSDI test, it states that it is reliable and its results are valid and reliable, it was performed on 132 people with a diagnosis of DES with an average age of 53 years [18]. In the present study, the OSDI test was used, to analyze the changes that occur after the sessions of IRPL. With respect to physical symptoms, the most prevalent was the sensation of a foreign body—grit, which was present almost all of the time, and the most frequent in daily activities was working in front of digital screens. Wind was the environmental factor that most affected the population. After the application of the PLRI, the symptoms decreased significantly, in agreement with the findings of the study by Miotto et al. [8], in which all 32 patients showed a decrease in the OSDI scale score.

The study conducted by Mejia et al. in 2019, in which they determined the effects of PLRI in 25 people with the use of visual symptom scales, determined the decrease in the score from an average of eight before the sessions to an average of three after the application of PLRI [19]. A research developed in Argentina in 2018, in order to describe the treatment and results obtained from the LPRRI in 100 cases of DES, used a scale from 1 to 10 that rated the health status perceived by the participants, before the treatment an average health score of seven was obtained and after the treatment it increased to eight [20].

3. Conclusions

- The majority of the patients were male, older than 58 years, with an average age of 56 years. Within the occupations, the most prevalent was found in the other category, which included: health personnel, drivers, engineers, and architects, followed by retirees.

- Regarding personal history, the most prevalent were arterial hypertension, thyroid diseases, diabetes mellitus, and Sjögren's syndrome, some of the patients presented more than one personal history. Among the ophthalmologic antecedents, cataracts, glaucoma, and pterygium were the most common.

- The most common symptoms in people treated at the Exiláser Ophthalmology Center were ocular pain, burning, photophobia, and foreign body sensation. The most characteristic signs were conjunctival hyperemesis and ocular dryness, followed by irregularity of the palpebral rim and blepharitis, which decreased after the IRPL sessions.

- The results showed improvement in glandular expression and decrease in pressure exerted, from severe to moderate intensity. Before treatment, granular glandular expression predominated and afterward nontransparent fluid prevailed, followed by clear transparent fluid.

- With the application of the OSDI test, it was found that the most common physical symptom during the day was foreign body sensation—grit, followed by photophobia. With respect to daily activities, the affectation was present during exposure to digital screens. Finally, the predominant environmental factor was the wind. After the application of the IRPL, the symptomatology decreased considerably.

Author details

Eduardo Rojas Alvarez[1]* and Naima Pino Urias[2]

1 Faculty of Medical Sciences, University of Cuenca, Ophthalmology in Exiláser Ophthalmological Center, Cuenca, Ecuador

2 French School of Cuenca, Ecuador

*Address all correspondence to: drerojasalvarez@gmail.com

References

[1] Shin KY, Lim DH, Moon CH, Kim BJ, Chung TY. Intense pulsed light plus meibomian gland expression versus intense pulsed light alone for meibomian gland dysfunction: A randomized crossover study. PLoS One. 2021;**16**(3):e0246245

[2] Rouen PA, White ML. Dry eye disease: Prevalence, assessment, and management. Home Healthcare Now. 2018;**36**(2):74-83

[3] Craig JP, Chen YH, Turnbull PRK. Prospective trial of intense pulsed light for the treatment of meibomian gland dysfunction. Investigative Ophthalmology & Visual Science. 2015;**56**(3):1965-1970

[4] Toyos R, McGill W, Briscoe D. Intense pulsed light treatment for dry eye disease due to meibomian gland dysfunction: A 3-Year Retrospective Study. Photomedicine and Laser Surgery. 2015;**33**(1):41-46

[5] Liu S, Tang S, Dong H, Huang X. Intense pulsed light for the treatment of Meibomian gland dysfunction: A systematic review and meta-analysis. Experimental and Therapeutic Medicine. 2020;**20**(2):1815-1821

[6] Cote S, Zhang AC, Ahmadzai V, Maleken A, Li C, Oppedisano J, et al. Intense pulsed light (IPL) therapy for the treatment of meibomian gland dysfunction. Cochrane Database System Review. 2020;**2020**(3):21. Disponible en: https://www.ncbi.nlm.nih.gov/pmc/articles/PMC7077992/

[7] Diburnet MS, Ruiz ACP, Ávila EG, Carvajal DD, Infante YP. Características epidemiológicas, clínicas y oftalmológicas de pacientes con queratoconjuntivitis seca. MEDISAN. 2021;**25**(6):1351-1360

[8] Miotto-Montesinos G, Rojas-Alvarez E, Torres-Piedra DM. Resultados preliminares del tratamiento con luz pulsada intensa regulada en el síndrome de ojo seco. RMO. 2019;**92**(6):1374

[9] Vergés C, Salgado-Borges J, Ribot FM de. Prospective evaluation of a new intense pulsed light, thermaeye plus, in the treatment of dry eye disease due to meibomian gland dysfunction. Journal of Optometry. 2021;14(2):103-113

[10] Dell SJ, Gaster RN, Barbarino SC, Cunningham DN. Prospective evaluation of intense pulsed light and meibomian gland expression efficacy on relieving signs and symptoms of dry eye disease due to meibomian gland dysfunction. Clinical Ophthalmology. 2017;**11**:817-827

[11] Tang Y, Liu R, Tu P, Song W, Qiao J, Yan X, et al. A Retrospective Study of treatment outcomes and prognostic factors of intense pulsed light therapy combined with meibomian gland expression in patients with meibomian gland dysfunction. Eye & Contact Lens. 2021;**47**(1):38-44

[12] Mendoza A, van der Goes TI F. Síndrome de ojo seco. Una revisión de la literatura. Rev Fac Med. 2021;**64**(5):46-54

[13] Shanti Y, Shehada R, Bakkar MM, Qaddumi J. Prevalence and associated risk factors of dry eye disease in 16 northern West bank towns in Palestine: a cross- sectional study. BMC Ophthalmology. 2020;**20**(1):26

[14] Armas Hernández A, Armengol Oramas Y, Alemán

Suárez I, Suárez Herrera V, Ribot Ruiz LA. Comportamiento clínico-oftalmológico del síndrome de ojo seco. Revista Médica Electrónica. 2018;**40**(1):81-88

[15] Pérez MV, Díaz de Alvarez C y P. Frecuencia de Ojo Seco y su Correlación con un Cuestionario Sintomatológico en Pacientes con Artritis Reumatoide. Revista de la Facultad de Medicina. 2001;**24**(2):145-150

[16] Merayo J, Benítez J, Montero J, Galarreta M, Alejandre A. Guías españolas para el tratamiento de la enfermedad de ojo seco. [Internet] 2017 [citado 20 de agosto de 2022]. Disponible en http://www.lasuperficieocular.com/resources/documents/guias_ojo_seco_SESOC_ THEA.pdf

[17] Garza-León M, Valencia-Garza M, Martínez-Leal B, Villarreal-Peña P, Marcos-Abdala HG, Cortéz-Guajardo AL, et al. Prevalence of ocular surface disease symptoms and risk factors in group of university students in Monterrey, Mexico. Journal of Ophthalmic Inflammation and Infection. 2016;**6**(1):44

[18] González J, Ulloa I, Correa O, Prieto L. Fiabilidad y Validez del Cuestionario OSDI (Ocular Disease Surface Index) en Pacientes con Diagnóstico de Síndrome de Ojo Seco en el Hospital Simón Bolívar. Colombia Review. 2015;**48**(3):262-276

[19] Mejía LF, Gil JC, Jaramillo M. Terapia de luz pulsada intensa regulada: un tratamiento complementario prometedor para la enfermedad de ojo seco. Archivos de la Sociedad Española de Oftalmología. 2019;**94**(7):331-336

[20] Cosentino MJ, Rodríguez C. Aplicación de luz pulsada intensa en el tratamiento del síndrome de ojo seco refractario al tratamiento clínico. 2019;7